Renal Disease: An Illustrated Guide

D. Gwyn Williams, MD, FRCP

Consultant Nephrologist and
Senior Lecturer in Medicine,
Guy's Hospital,
London

Published,
in association with
UPDATE PUBLICATIONS LTD., by

MTP PRESS LIMITED
International Medical Publishers

Published,
in association with
Update Publications Ltd., by

MTP Press Limited
Falcon House
Lancaster, England

Softcover reprint of the hardcover 1st edition 1981

First published 1981

ISBN-13: 978-94-009-8068-6 e-ISBN-13: 978-94-009-8066-2
DOI: 10.1007/978-94-009-8066-2

Contents

Preface

This book does not pretend to be a comprehensive textbook of nephrology, nor is it a guide to the management of renal disease, as space does not allow the description or discussion of investigation and treatment.

Its intention is to illustrate the diverse diseases which present to nephrologists. Since the key to understanding the effects and progression of a disease are to know and comprehend its pathology, I have approached the subject not by discussing presenting symptoms of single diseases in different sections, which would lead to much repetition, but by describing the disorders according to the mechanisms which cause them. To illustrate the text I have chosen the most immediate clue which usually appears in a given disease, which may therefore be a clinical sign, a radiograph or the histological appearance of a renal biopsy.

D. Gwyn Williams
Guy's Hospital, London

1. Trauma

Trauma is a common cause of acute renal failure. This may arise directly from injuries to the kidneys themselves despite their protected position (Figure 1). Trauma can also cause acute renal failure by damaging the renal arteries, which may be actually avulsed from the kidneys, or stretched at the time of impact, with tearing of the arterial wall and secondary thrombosis. Figure 2 shows the renal arteriogram of a young man who presented with anuric acute renal failure after a motorbike accident. Only the upper pole of the right kidney is

Figure 1. *IVU showing extravasated contrast (arrowed) and nephrectomy specimen of ruptured kidney following a road accident.*

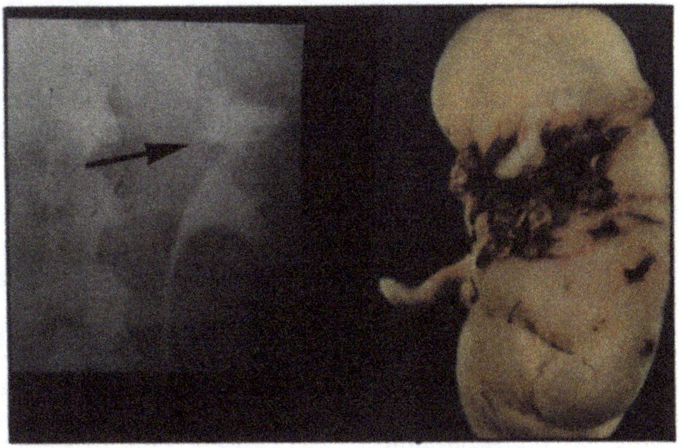

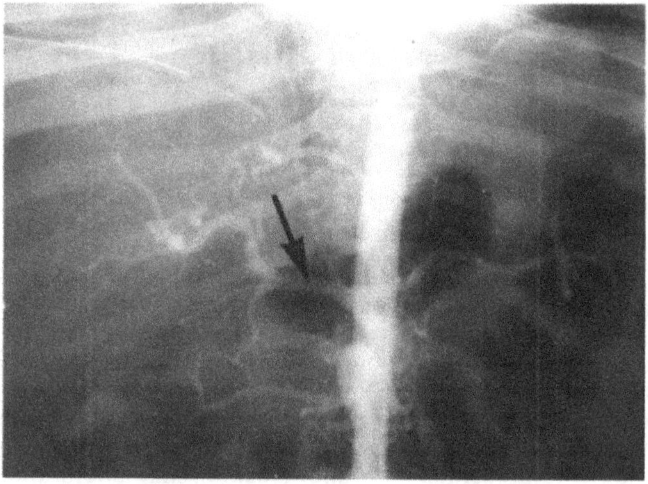

Figure 2. *Arteriogram of patient with acute renal failure following road accident showing occlusion of two left renal arteries and lower of two right renal arteries and an upper right renal artery which is patent (arrowed).*

perfused since this patient had two renal arteries to each kidney, and only one remains patent. The renal veins may be similarly avulsed, also causing acute renal failure.

Pelvic or abdominal injuries can cause acute renal failure by producing obstruction to or loss of continuity of the outflow tract. Trauma also contributes to renal failure by producing myoglobinaemia, myoglobinuria and fat emboli, which may also affect the brain, lungs and skin (Figure 3). Surgical operations are a refined form of trauma and the rare mistake of accidental ureteric ligation should never be forgotten as a possible cause of postoperative renal failure.

Acute renal failure due to trauma occurs most frequently through the indirect effect of fluid loss, e.g. in haemorrhage, or burns (Figure 4). Postoperative fluid and electrolyte loss can also lead to acute renal failure, but this is preventable by appropriate management.

Figure 3. *Purpura due to fat emboli in the skin.*

Figure 4. *Severe burns causing acute renal failure.*

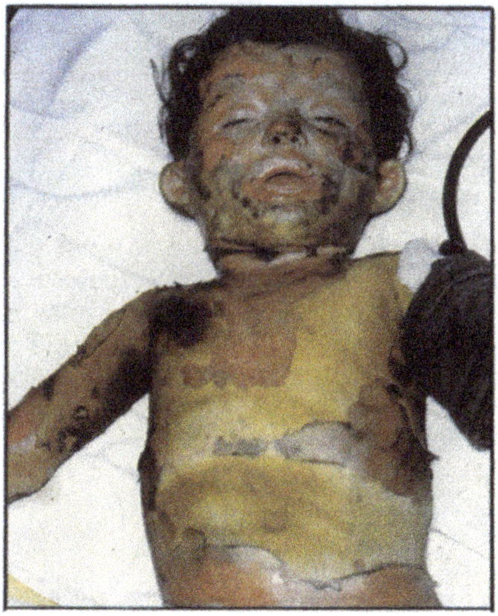

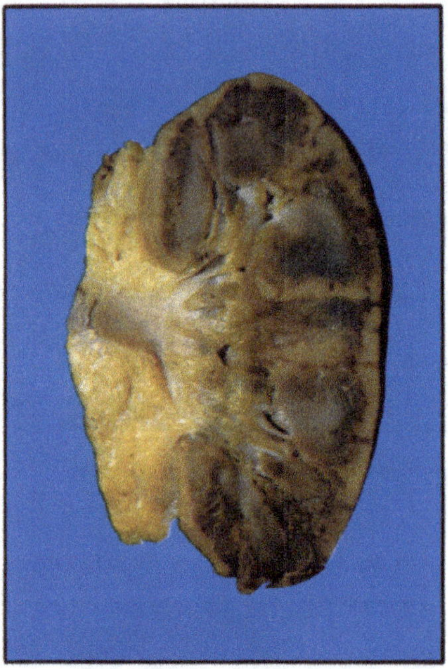

Figure 5. *Cortical necrosis following postpartum haemorrhage and acute renal failure.*

If the patient survives traumatic acute renal failure, then for practical purposes renal function recovers completely. Occasionally injury causes long-term renal disease, for example, cortical necrosis (Figure 5). Chronic renal failure may also result from obstruction, following injury to the outflow tract, or from ischaemia and hypertension due to damaged renal vessels.

2. Infections

Urinary tract infections are described in a separate book in this series (Walls 1981) and will not be considered here. Systemic infections can affect the kidney; these are described according to the organisms responsible.

Bacterial Infections

The most important renal effect of a bacterial infection is septicaemic acute renal failure caused by several factors, i.e. shock, endotoxinaemia, and disseminated intravascular coagulation. This usually follows trauma, or major surgery with postoperative care necessitating multiple invasion of the patient's normally intact skin and mucosal defences. Less commonly the cause is a primary bacterial infection, e.g. peritonitis, streptococcal or staphylococcal septicaemia (Figure 6). Rarely the kidney itself is colonized by the invading organisms. On nephro-urological wards it is worth remembering the dangers of injudicious urethral catheterization; in particular it is futile to catheterize the oliguric or anuric non-obstructed patient for a prolonged period in order to record the passage of little or no urine.

Large single or multiple abscesses in or around the kidney are important treatable postludes to bacterial infections. Patients present with fever, loin pain, occasionally pyuria and haematuria, and septicaemia recurring from the abscess itself (Figure 7).

Prolonged bacterial infections may cause renal disease by an entirely different pathogenetic mechanism. Thus, bacterial endocarditis and chronic infection of atrioventricular shunts present the body with a persistent antigen, and consequently immune complex glomerulonephritis develops (see page 50).

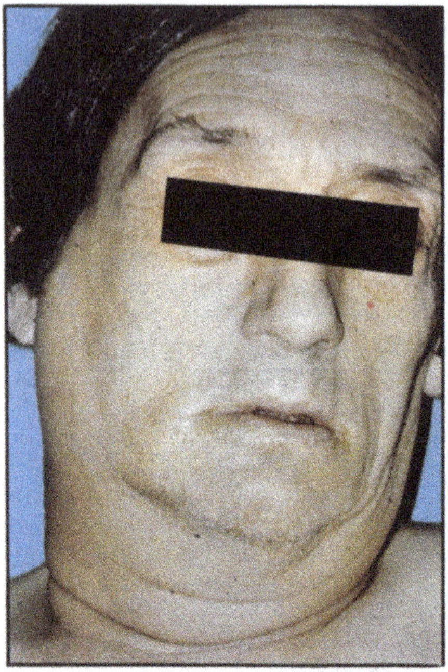

Figure 6. *Staphylococcal parotitis leading to staphylococcal septicaemia and acute renal failure.*

Viral Infections

Apart from immunosuppressed transplanted patients who may suffer from cytomegalovirus infection of the kidney, direct viral invasion of renal tissue is an extremely rare cause of disease. On the other hand, mumps, measles, hepatitis, and EB virus have all been implicated as causes of immune complex glomerulonephritis with varying degrees of proof ranging from mere association to demonstration of the virus and its antibody in the kidney.

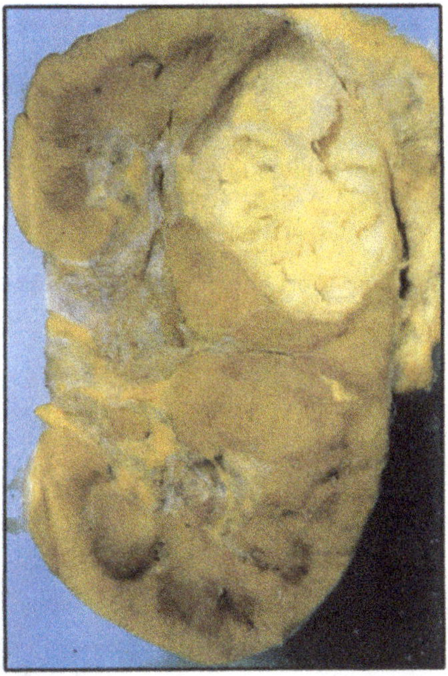

Figure 7. *Renal abscess.*

Other Infections

Malaria. This is famous for causing blackwater fever, an uncommon event following infection with *Plasmodium falciparum*. The renal involvement is a result of the haemolysis and disseminated intravascular coagulation compounded by shock.

Quartan malaria (*Plasmodium malariae*) in Uganda and Nigeria is associated with a nephrotic syndrome due to an immune complex with the parasite as antigen.

Leptospirosis. Leptospira icterohaemorrhagiae and to a lesser extent *Leptospira canicola* can cause acute renal failure. The patient frequently has a history of exposure to sites where rats are found, e.g. rivers, old buildings, farms. Infection with *Leptospira icterohaemorrhagiae* is characterized by severe jaundice, frequently with disproportionately less severe abnormalities in other liver function tests, and conjunctival injection (Figure 8).

Schistosomiasis. Schistosoma haematobium is a major cause of death and morbidity in the Middle East by its infec-

Figure 8. *Jaundice and conjunctivitis in a man with leptospirosis.*

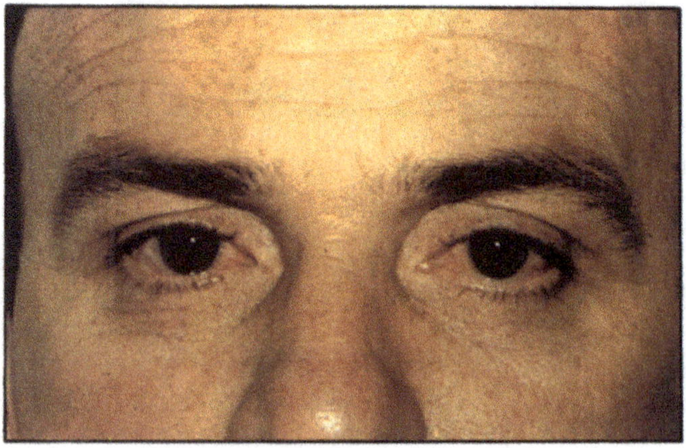

tion of the bladder and ureters, with consequent contraction and deformity of the bladder, ureteric stricture and hydronephrosis (Figure 9). Patients present with haematuria, dysuria and renal failure. The risk of carcinoma of the bladder is increased. Schistosomal infections have also been alleged to cause nephritis.

Syphilis. A nephrotic syndrome occurs in both congenital and secondary syphilis as a result of an immune complex glomerulonephritis. It is important to be aware of this diagnosis as the response to specific therapy is often good.

Fungal infections. Colonization of the urinary tract by *Candida* species occasionally occurs in patients with poor immune defences due to drugs or severe illness, or in patients who have had prolonged intubation of some part of their urinary tract. Rarely a mycetoma may form and give rise to the added complication of obstruction.

Figure 9. *Plain radiograph showing vesical and ureteric calcification due to schistosomiasis.*

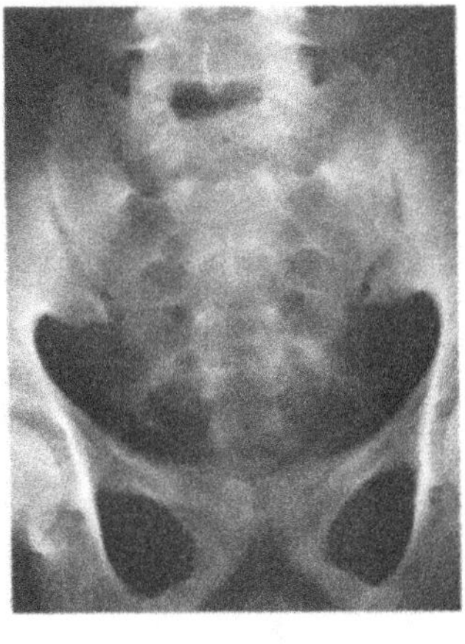

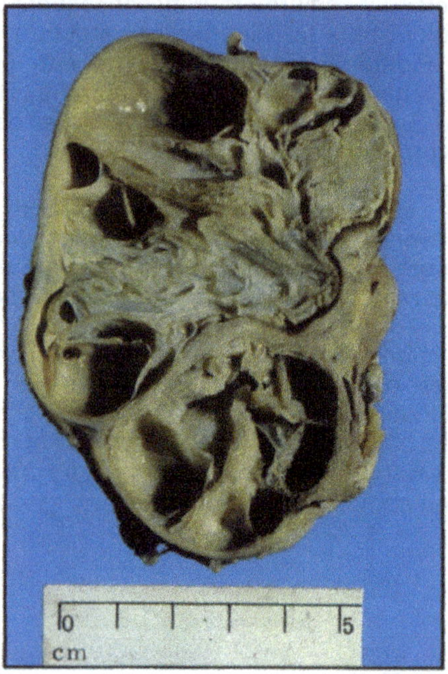

Figure 10. *Hydatid cysts in kidney.*

Hydatid disease. Infection with *Echinococcus* (*granulosus* and *multilocularis*) causes cyst formation affecting the brain, liver, spleen and kidney (Figure 10). Hydatid disease is found in sheep farming areas, and patients may be asymptomatic or present with haematuria, loin pain and swelling, and symptoms due to involvement of other organs.

3. Neoplasms

The kidneys may be affected in several ways by tumours; they may be the site of neoplasia, obstruction to the urinary tract may occur, tumours may secrete hormones which alter renal function, neoplasms may cause renal vein thrombosis, hyperuricaemia or hypercalcaemia may complicate malignancy, and glomerulonephritis may result from immune complexes of tumour antigen and antibody.

Neoplasia in the Kidney

Adenomas are the commonest benign tumour and are usually silent. Hamartomas are associated with tuberous sclerosis and may present with haemorrhage and pain, or may be detected when the patient develops fits or presents with mental retardation and the typical facial adenoma sebaceum (Figure 11).

Malignant tumours usually cause haematuria and loin pain, which may be associated with fever in the case of hypernephroma. This tumour (renal cell carcinoma, Grawitz's tumour) is the commonest primary malignant growth of the kidney; others are the carcinomas of the collecting system and nephroblastoma (Wilm's tumour) in childhood. Abdominal enlargement may be the first feature noted in the latter (Figure 12). The diagnosis of nephroblastoma has become particularly important because in recent years the prognosis has improved considerably.

Other neoplasms may involve the kidneys by infiltration. The commonest example with clinical consequences is myeloma, which can damage the kidney in several ways. The

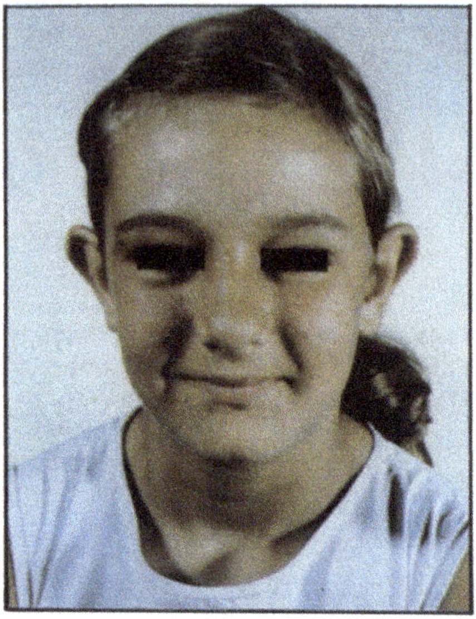

Figure 11. *Tuberous sclerosis.*

Figure 12. *Abdominal enlargement due to Wilm's tumour.*

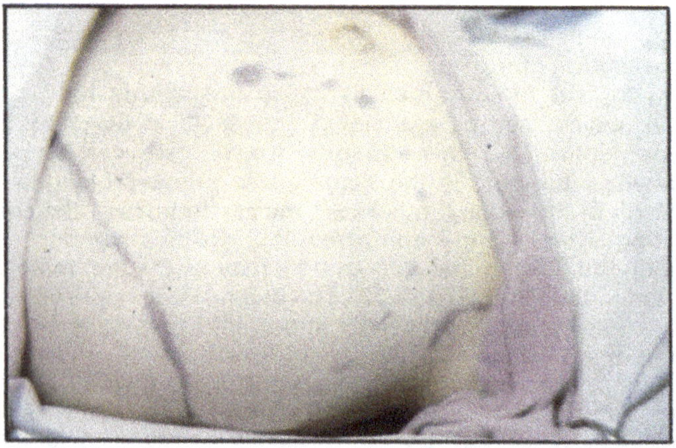

plasma cells may infiltrate the kidney to produce structural damage, although some of the functional effects of the infiltration are reversible by treatment. The abnormal protein may actually deposit in the tubules. Hypercalcaemia or hyperuricaemia may occur in myeloma, and these may cause renal damage. Finally, the kidney may develop amyloid or a plasmacytoma.

The combination of infiltration and tubular protein deposition can cause acute renal failure. Myeloma should be considered as a cause of acute renal failure if the kidneys appear larger than normal radiographically (presumably due to the infiltration). Figure 13 shows the IVU of a patient who presented with a two-month history of malaise preceding acute renal failure. The other dysproteinaemia which may involve the kidneys is Waldenstrom's macroglobulinaemia. Leukaemias and the lymphomas may also infiltrate the renal parenchyma, but this is a rare clinical complication.

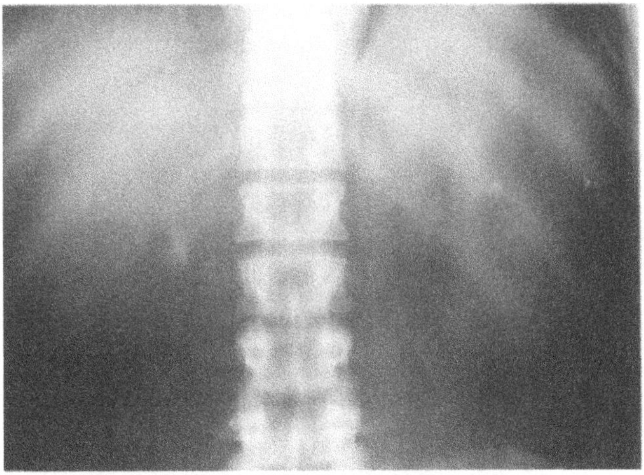

Figure 13. *IVU of patient with renal failure due to myeloma, showing bilateral diffuse enlargement of the kidneys.*

Amyloid is not conventionally regarded as a neoplasm, but it represents uncontrolled production of protein molecules by plasma cells, which may themselves be proliferating. Primary amyloid is characterized by deposition of amyloid, consisting of portions of immunoglobulin light chains. Amyloid of similar characteristics and distribution occurs in myeloma, macroglobulinaemia and lymphomas. Secondary amyloid, which develops in rheumatoid arthritis, chronic infections (tuberculosis, osteomyelitis and bronchiectasis), ulcerative colitis, regional ileitis and familial mediterranean fever consists of amyloid associated (AA) protein which is distinguishable from immunoglobulins.

The patient may present with proteinuria, nephrotic syndrome or chronic renal failure plus complaints due to involvement of other organs. Figures 14 and 15 illustrate a case in which the chronic infection had arisen in the kidney itself. The patient presented with a nephrotic syndrome and discharge of pus from the right thigh. Twenty-six years

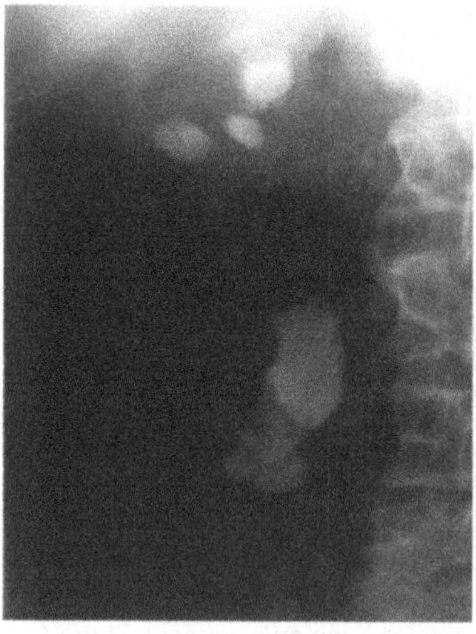

Figure 14. *Plain radiograph showing staghorn calculus and cortical calculi in a patient with amyloidosis.*

earlier he had had a right pyelolithotomy, following which there had been a chronic purulent discharge from different areas over the right loin. Right nephrectomy revealed a chronic perirenal abscess around a destroyed kidney containing a staghorn calculus.

Obstruction

Tumours obstructing urinary outflow may result in acute or chronic renal failure. Usually such tumours are of the prostate, bladder (Figures 16, 17), cervix, and less commonly ureters, pelvis of the kidney or rectum. Retroperitoneal

Figure 15. *Sinuses in same patient as Figure 14.*

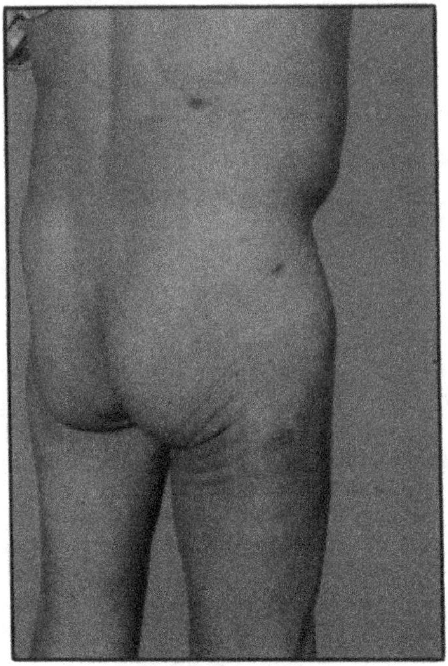

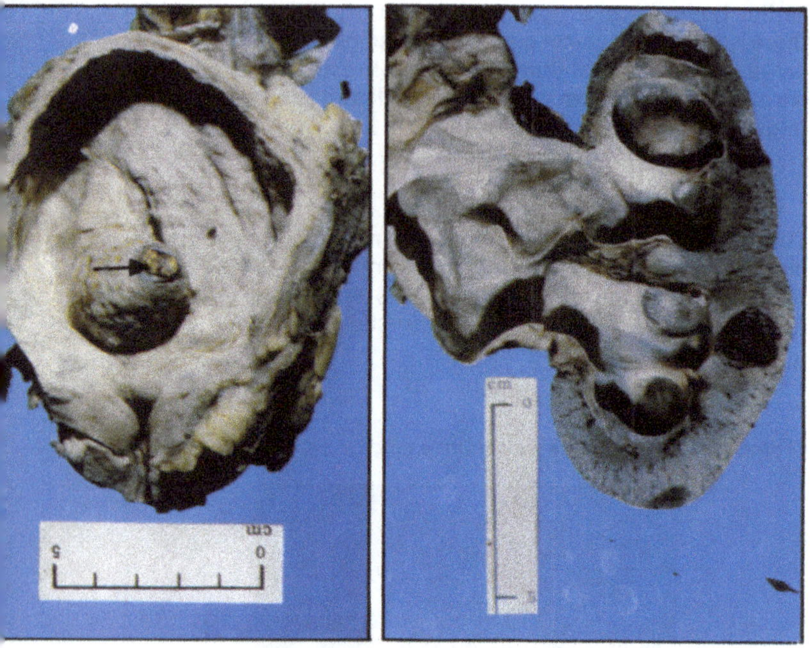

Figures 16 and 17. *Carcinoma of the bladder involving ureteric orifice (arrowed left) causing hydroureter and hydronephrosis (right). (N.B. The left-hand figure is the right way up even though the measure is inverted.)*

lymphomata can cause obstruction by compression and involvement of the ureters. In retroperitoneal fibrosis (malignant in approximately 10 per cent of cases), firm, dense, fibrous tissue obstructs the ureters, usually without compressing them. This tissue may extend to involve the inferior vena cava, the common bile duct and the mediastinum. The urinary symptoms are sometimes characterized by a 'stop–go' pattern of oliguria and anuria interspersed with polyuria, and patients also frequently complain of back pain. Radiology demonstrates the distorted course and irregular lumen of the ureter (Figure 18).

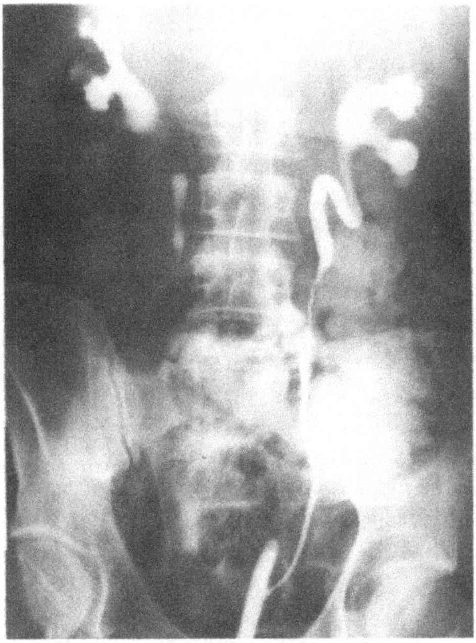

Figure 18. *Retrograde urography in retroperitoneal fibrosis.*

Neoplasia and Glomerulonephritis

Antigens implicated in human immune complex nephritis include those expressed on the surface of malignant cells. These neoplasms causing nephritis occur most commonly in the lung, but cases of carcinoma of the ovary, the prostate, the kidney itself and the stomach have all been described. Figure 19 shows a Horner's syndrome in a patient who presented with a nephrotic syndrome. The histology in these carcinoma-associated nephropathies is membranous glomerulonephritis, and 10 per cent of patients with this form of nephritis have malignant disease.

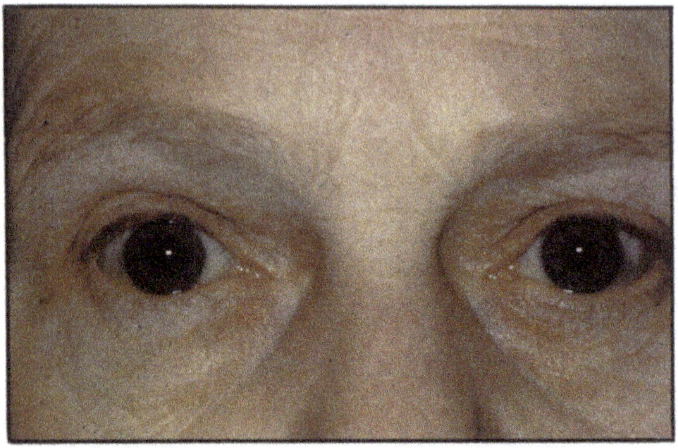

Figure 19. *Horner's syndrome in a patient with nephrotic syndrome due to membranous nephropathy associated with carcinoma of the lung.*

Hodgkin's disease (Figure 20) may be complicated by a nephrotic syndrome in which glomerular histology shows a 'minimal change' appearance. The nature of this relationship is unclear, and is likely to remain so in view of our current ignorance of the pathogenesis of minimal change nephrotic syndrome.

The connection between malignant disease and nephritis is of further interest because the glomerular lesion can improve with removal or suppression of the neoplasm, presumably, in the case of the immune complex type of membranous nephritis, as a result of removal of the antigen.

Neoplasia and Ectopic Hormone Production

Tumours may contain dedifferentiated cells which produce hormones or peptides chemically and functionally similar to hormones. Some of these substances, such as parathyroid hormone and ACTH, may have profound effects on the kidneys.

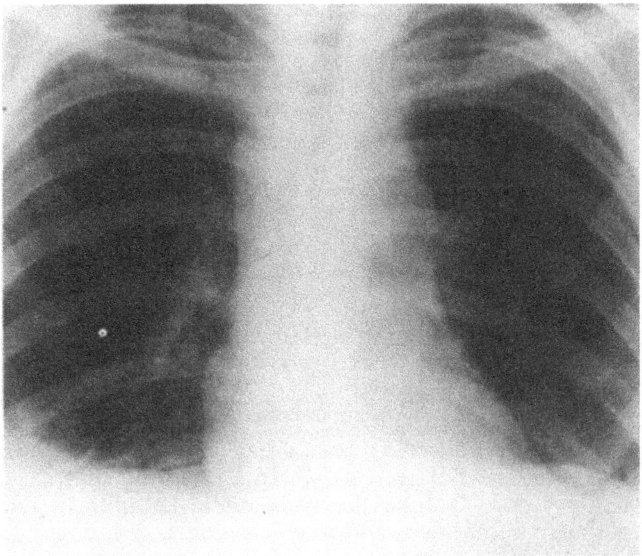

Figure 20. *Bilateral hilar lymphadenopathy due to Hodgkin's disease in a patient presenting with nephrotic syndrome.*

Hypercalcaemia and Hyperuricaemia

See Chapter 6.

Renal Vein Thrombosis

Extrinsic pressure on the renal vein by tumour, direct invasion of its lumen, and a nephrotic syndrome secondary to amyloidosis or membranous nephropathy may all result in renal vein thrombosis.

4. Vascular Disease

Several disorders may affect the renal blood vessels with consequent disease of the kidney itself.

Hypertension

Chronic high blood pressure is the cause of terminal renal failure in seven per cent of patients receiving dialysis or transplantation. Despite the well-known benefits of anti-hypertensive treatment and the more effective and less unpleasant drugs now available, nephrologists commonly see patients with end stage renal disease due to neglected or mismanaged hypertension.

Accelerated or malignant hypertension, which can arise seemingly de novo or in a patient with recognized hypertension, is renowned for its rapid and devastating effects on the brain and the kidney. Patients may exhibit a wide range of clinical features: at one extreme they may be virtually asymptomatic but referred for control of hypertension and at the other they present with fits and coma. The clinical hallmark is the retinopathy, comprising papilloedema, haemorrhages and exudates, and this may lead to blindness (Figure 21). The pathological hallmark is the necrotizing lesion with fibrin deposition in the walls of small arteries and arterioles which results in ischaemia and infarction of the organ or tissue supplied. The changes in the small vessels can also lead to the consumption of platelets and local destruction of erythrocytes causing thrombocytopenia and microangiopathic haemolytic anaemia.

Accelerated hypertension carries a high morbidity, with the possibility of permanent damage to brain, eyes, heart

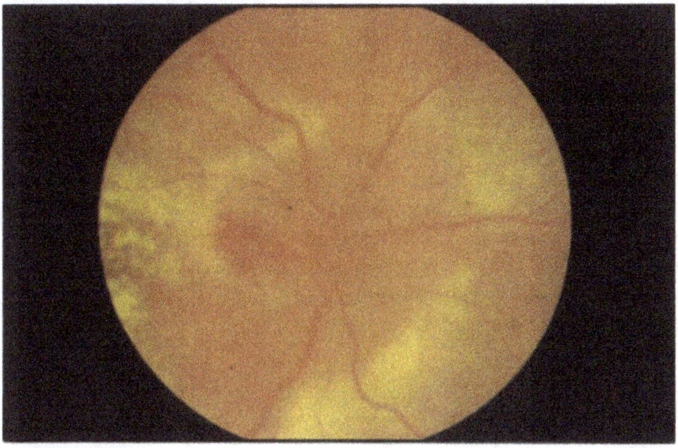

Figure 21. *Papilloedema, haemorrhage and exudates in a 28-year-old woman with accelerated hypertension and terminal renal failure.*

and kidneys, and a high mortality. These consequences can be modified or prevented by prompt treatment, depending on the initial state of the patient. A small proportion of patients who present with renal failure severe enough to require dialysis regain renal function which, although impaired, is adequate for independent survival.

Renal Artery Stenosis

The clinical features indicating this diagnosis are the tendency to occur in younger patients, lack of family history and recent onset of hypertension. The patient may have noted loin pain and occasional haematuria indicating that infarction has occurred; polyuria is rare. A renal artery bruit may be heard. In unilateral disease intravenous urography shows that the affected kidney is smaller than the healthier kidney, with delayed excretion on early films and a denser nephrogram on later films.

The cause of the arterial narrowing is usually a plaque of atheroma or thrombosis, and less commonly is an embolus which has not produced complete occlusion. Rarer causes are external compression of the renal artery by tumours or cysts, and fibromuscular dysplasia of the arterial wall. The latter is a condition in which the muscle coat of the renal arteries is hypertrophied, producing luminal narrowing and a tortuous vessel (Figure 22). This condition tends to affect young adults, particularly females. It is sometimes associated with arterial abnormalities of other organs, particularly brain and spleen, haemorrhage into which may be the presenting feature. Fibromuscular dysplasia has been related to Takayashu's disease, which itself may involve the renal arteries.

Thrombosis

Arterial

Thrombi in the renal arteries usually form on a plaque of atheroma; less commonly they are related to intimal damage following trauma or operations. They may cause infarction when complete, and hypertension when incomplete. In a few patients renal artery thrombosis leads to chronic and progressive renal failure. This is of practical importance, since removing or bypassing the thrombosis alleviates the renal failure. The clinical pointers are progressive renal failure in a patient of the right age group, possibly accompanied by hypertension, by vascular disease affecting other organs, by unequal size of the kidneys on intravenous urography and, if repeat radiographic examinations are made, by the kidney(s) becoming smaller. Arteriography proves the diagnosis (Figure 23).

Venous

Renal vein thrombosis is a serious complication of the nephrotic syndrome (Figure 24);it is rarely a primary event leading to the nephrotic syndrome. The blood of a nephrotic patient is hypercoagulable owing to the increased concentrations of factors VII and VIII.

The clinical onset of renal vein thrombosis is usually insidious, and since its effects are proteinuria with or without haematuria, it may go unnoticed against the background of

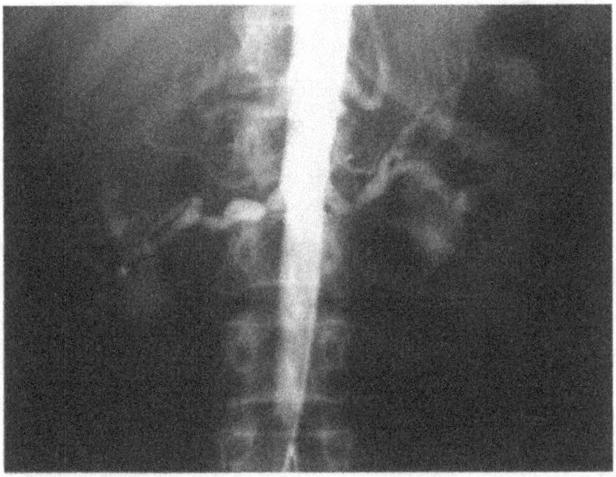

Figure 22. *Renal arteriogram showing fibromuscular dysplasia in a 24-year-old woman with hypertension.*

Figure 23. *Early phase arteriogram showing left renal artery stenosis (encircled) in a middle-aged woman with severe hypertension.*

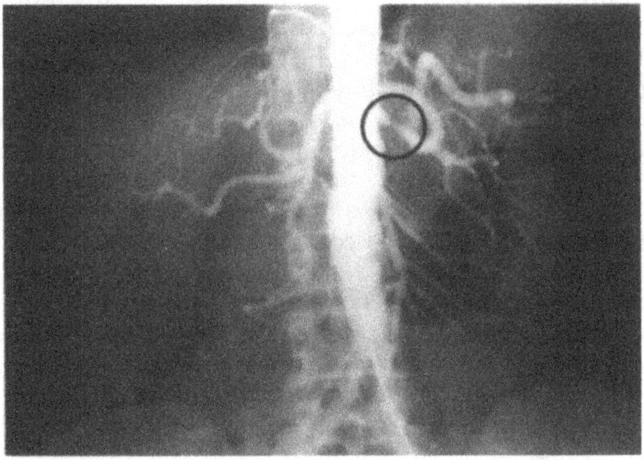

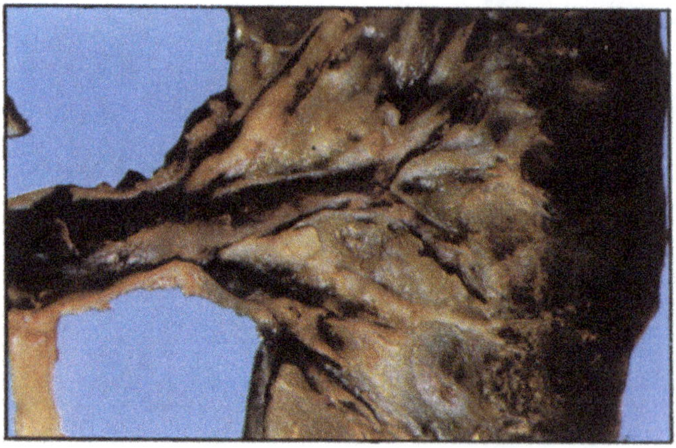

Figure 24. *Renal vein thrombosis in a 58-year-old woman who had a nephrotic syndrome due to membranous nephropathy.*

the nephrotic syndrome itself. Warning signs are the worsening of proteinuria and hypoproteinaemia, oedema requiring greater doses of diuretics, falling renal function, and, in minimal change nephrotic syndrome, failure to respond to steroid therapy. Occasionally the thrombosis occurs acutely with loin pain, macroscopic haematuria and acute renal failure. Sites other than the renal veins may thrombose in the nephrotic syndrome (e.g. the inferior vena cava, and the cavernous sinus). As with any venous thrombosis, pulmonary emboli may occur as complications.

Renal vein thrombosis as a primary event causing a nephrotic syndrome or acute renal failure occurs particularly in severely dehydrated children. It may also complicate tumours within the kidney, extrinsic pressure on the renal veins by tumours or abnormal renal arteries, trauma to the renal vessels, and primary venous thrombosis in the pelvis and abdomen.

Emboli

The commonest sources of renal emboli are mural thrombosis after a myocardial infarction, and vegetations on diseased heart valves. The consequence of a large embolus affecting the main artery or one of its larger branches is infarction and, should the embolus be infected, an abscess may follow and, rarely, a mycotic aneurysm. Clinically a major embolus may be silent, present with loin pain with or without haematuria, and, in the case of bilateral emboli, can give rise to acute renal failure.

Microemboli occur as a complication of mitral stenosis, and these have been implicated in the hypertension accompanying this disease. Fat emboli are a complication of trauma.

Atheroma

Atheroma of the renal arteries has already been mentioned; it may result in hypertension, chronic renal failure or infarction.

Vasculitis

Polyarteritis

Vasculitis affecting the kidney involves the renal arteries and not the veins, and therefore this term is used interchangeably with polyarteritis. The major renal arteries are infrequently involved in polyarteritis nodosa; when they are, renal failure with or without infarction may ensue (Figure 25). More frequently vasculitis affects the kidneys in microscopic polyarteritis. The vessels involved range from the interlobular to those of the glomerular tuft, and the glomeruli typically exhibit a segmental fibrinoid necrosis with crescents. Clinical evidence of arteritis elsewhere is uncommon, but at postmortem arteritis may be demonstrable in the adrenals, testis, spleen or lung (Figure 26). The patients are middle-aged to elderly, and often complain of malaise, arthralgia and fever. Examination may reveal no abnormalities, but some patients have a vasculitic rash (Figure 27), which in some cases is suggestive of Henoch–Schönlein purpura and, more

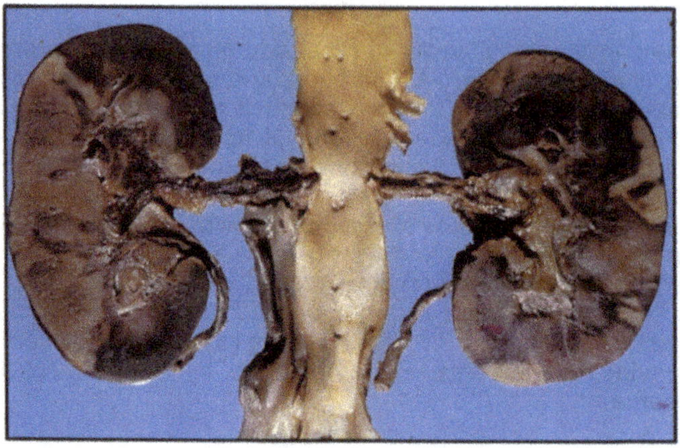

Figure 25. *Bilateral renal artery thrombosis in a patient with polyarteritis nodosa.*

Figure 26. *Small artery in lung with fibrinoid necrosis and obliteration of its lumen (MSB stain, × 60).*

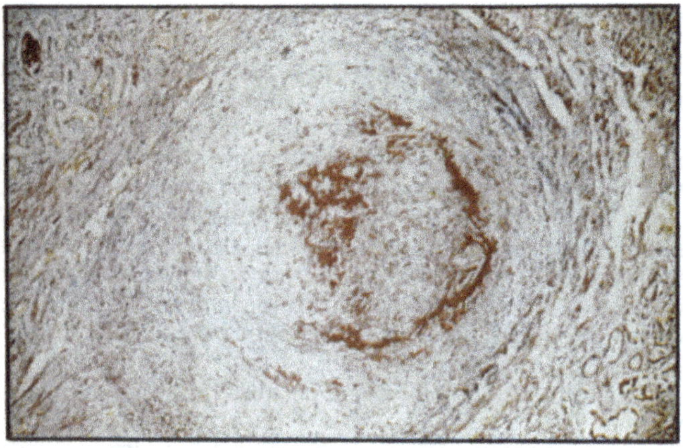

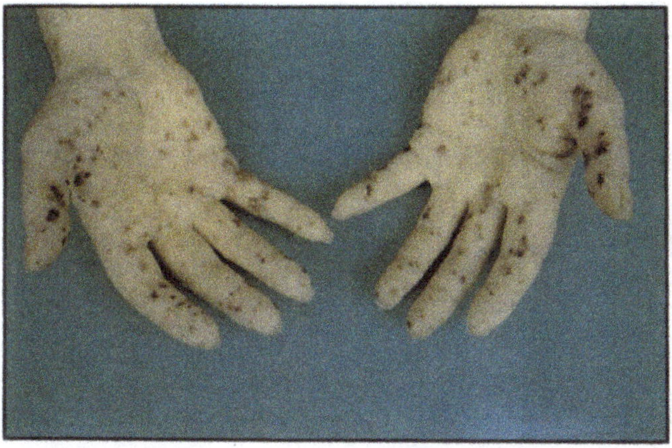

Figure 27. *Vasculitic rash on hands of 72-year-old man with acute renal failure due to microscopic polyarteritis.*

characteristically, a few patients have small infarcts in the nail folds of the hands (Figure 28) or feet. Most patients present with renal impairment, frequently severe and rapidly deteriorating. The diagnosis is important, as treatment (with immunosuppression with or without anticoagulants) seems to halt or reverse the disease with a survival rate of approximately 50 per cent.

Wegener's Granulomatosis

An arteritis histologically similar to polyarteritis may affect the renal arteries in patients with Wegener's granulomatosis. The renal disease may be the overwhelming presenting feature and seemingly minor complaints, such as epistaxis, nasal stuffiness and cough, may be overlooked. Lesions of the nasal, pharyngeal, tracheal and bronchial mucosa may be present, and a chest radiograph may reveal pulmonary lesions (Figure 29).

Henoch–Schönlein Purpura

Henoch–Schönlein purpura is characterized pathologically by a vasculitis involving the skin, gastrointestinal tract,

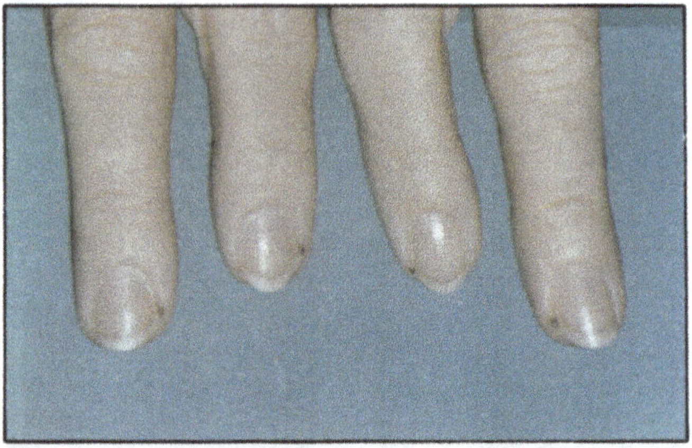

Figure 28. *Nail-fold infarcts in fingers of both hands in a 52-year-old woman with microscopic polyarteritis.*

Figure 29. *Chest radiograph showing pulmonary opacities in a patient with acute renal failure due to microscopic polyarteritis in Wegener's granulomatosi.*

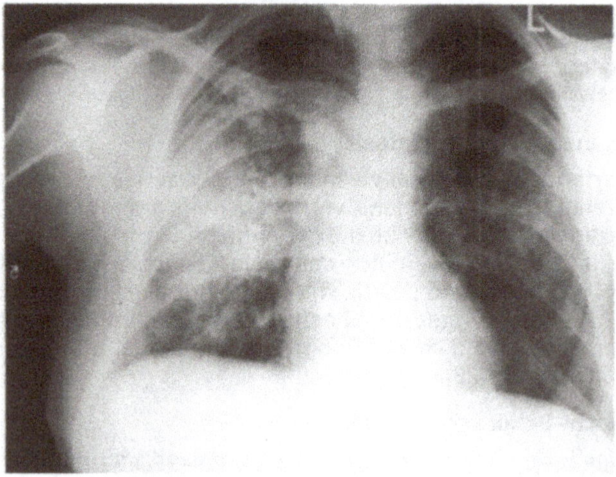

kidney and occasionally brain, and by a glomerulonephritis typically of a mesangioproliferative type (Figure 30). The tell-tale purpuric rash on the buttocks and extensor limb surfaces (Figure 31), with an accompanying arthralgia in most cases, makes the diagnosis. Not infrequently the rash has disappeared by the time the renal disease is severe enough to warrant the attention of a nephrologist, making the clinical diagnosis more difficult. In the acute attack evidence of renal involvement is found in 30 to 60 per cent of cases, depending on the referral pattern. The majority of cases of nephritis regress, but it is now apparent that a major complication of Henoch–Schönlein purpura is progressive renal disease terminating in chronic renal failure. There is no correlation between this and the severity of the acute attack.

SLE and Scleroderma

Arteritis of the renal vessels also occurs in systemic lupus erythematosus and scleroderma.

Figure 30. *Mesangial cell proliferation in a patient with Henoch–Schönlein purpura (H and E stain, × 250).*

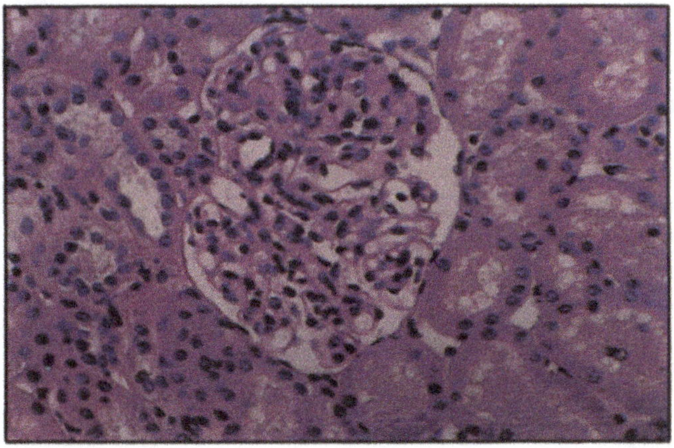

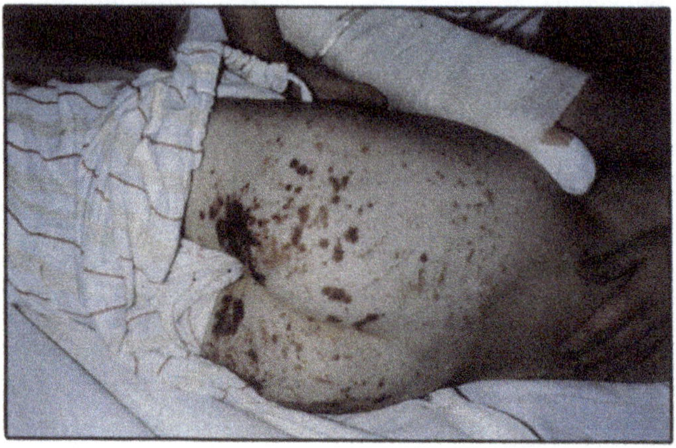

Figure 31. *Typical rash in a boy with Henoch–Schönlein purpura who had glomerulonephritis.*

5. Intravascular Disorders

The term intravascular disorders refers to diseases affecting platelets, erythrocytes and the clotting system, associated with renal damage.

Haemolytic Uraemic Syndrome

The haemolytic uraemic syndrome was originally described in children who, following a respiratory or gastrointestinal infection, became ill with oliguria, uraemia, haemolytic anaemia and thrombocytopenia. Bleeding, particularly from the gastrointestinal tract, and purpura occur, and occasionally there is neurological involvement. A similar picture has been recognized in adults following infection and pregnancy, and in women taking oral contraceptives.

In addition to thrombocytopenia and microangiopathic haemolytic anaemia (Figure 32), coagulation is abnormal; the thrombin time is prolonged and fibrin degradation products are increased. The disseminated intravascular coagulation is responsible for the fibrin deposition and the thrombi found in the arteries and arterioles of affected organs.

Many childhood cases recover, but in some cases there remains a tendency to develop hypertension and impaired renal function. The prognosis for recovery of renal function in adults is less good.

Disseminated Intravascular Coagulation

Apart from presenting as part of the haemolytic uraemic syndrome, disseminated intravascular coagulation occurs with renal involvement in septicaemia, accelerated hypertension and toxaemia of pregnancy. The lesions in affected

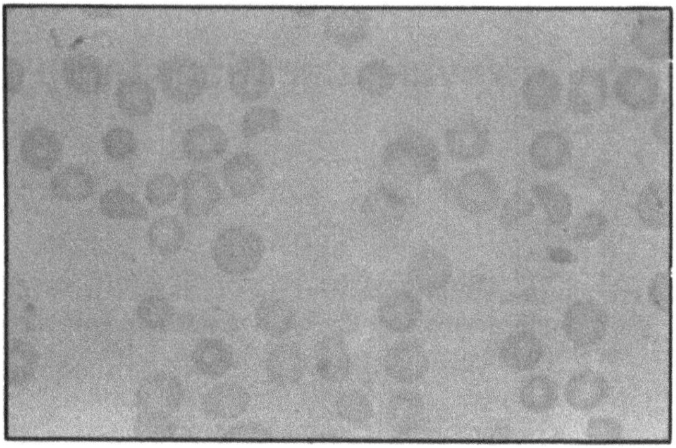

Figure 32. *Blood film showing distorted and fragmented erythrocytes from a child with haemolytic uraemic syndrome.*

organs arise from intravascular platelet aggregation and fibrin deposition, which cause the associated intravascular microangiopathic haemolytic anaemia (Figures 33 and 34).

Thrombotic thrombocytopenic purpura (Moschowitz's disease) is a related condition also characterized by purpura, bleeding, thrombocytopenia and microangiopathic haemolytic anaemia. Its original description emphasized the lesions of the central nervous system, which may be intermittent, and its occurrence in young adults, usually females. It is probably best regarded as an idiopathic form of disseminated intravascular coagulation and a variant of the haemolytic uraemic syndrome.

Intravascular Haemolysis

Severe haemolysis, e.g. as in mismatched transfusions or malaria, can cause acute renal failure. Haemoglobin itself is not toxic, but vasoconstrictive substances are released from the damaged erythrocyte membrane.

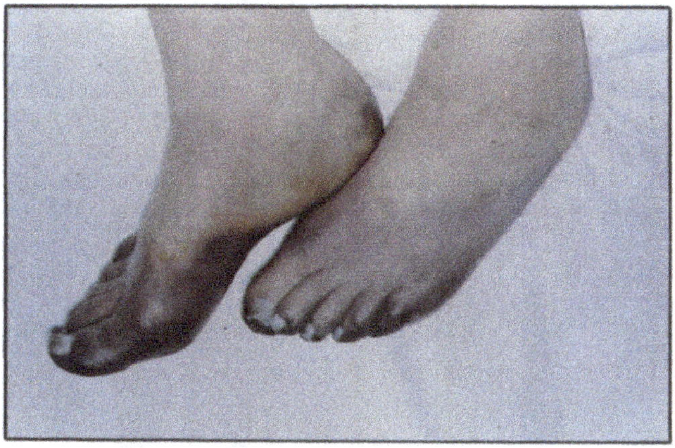

Figure 33. *Infarction of toes and feet in a man with Gram negative septicaemia.*

Figure 34. *Thrombosis in small vessel in interstitial tissue of testis, from patient with disseminated intravascular coagulation (MSB stain, × 400).*

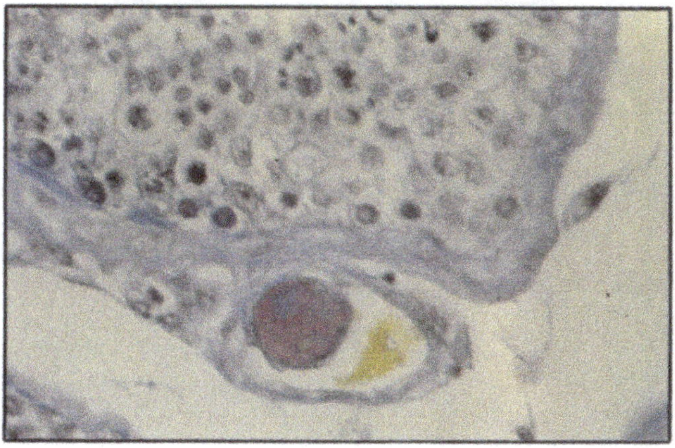

Sickle Cell Disease

Sickle cell disease affects approximately one in 700 Negroes. Patients present with haematuria (which also occurs in sickle cell trait), renal infarction, papillary necrosis, and rarely a glomerulopathy which can cause a nephrotic syndrome. These complaints may be seen against a background of other effects of sickle cell disease such as joint pains, leg ulcers (Figure 35), abdominal pains, failure to grow and anaemia.

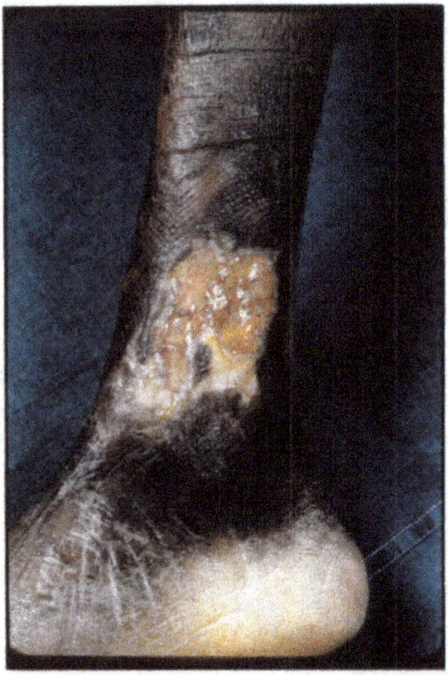

Figure 35. *Ulceration of lateral aspect of lower leg in sickle cell disease.*

6. Metabolic Disorders

Hypercalcaemia

Hypercalcaemia may affect the kidney by stone formation, nephrocalcinosis (in which there are multiple small intrarenal deposits of calcium with a distinctive radiological appearance (Figure 36)) or a reduction of kidney function and parenchymal loss without gross evidence of calcium deposition. Any of the causes of hypercalcaemia may be responsible, e.g. hyperparathyroidism, sarcoidosis, excess vitamin D, idiopathic hypercalcaemia of children and malignancy.

Figure 36. *Plain abdominal radiograph showing nephrocalcinosis.*

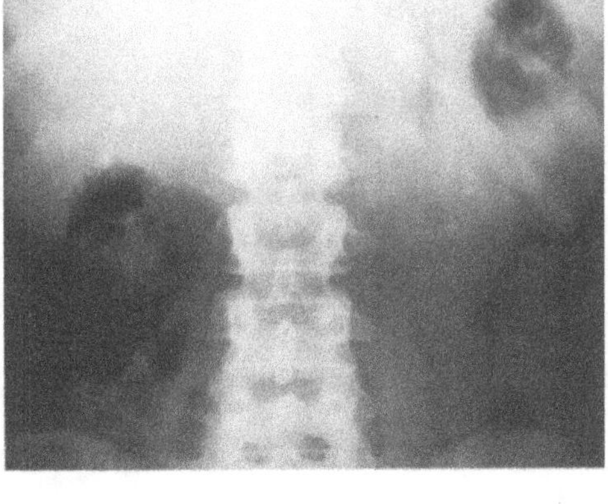

Stone formation, however, does not occur in neoplastic hypercalcaemia, as the metabolic abnormality is not sufficiently prolonged.

Therefore hypercalcaemic patients may present with any of the symptoms of renal stones and renal failure, as well as with complaints attributable to the primary disease and to hypercalcaemia itself—thirst, polydipsia, polyuria, peptic ulceration, acute pancreatitis, mental disorders and weakness. Acute renal failure is sometimes caused by acute hypercalcaemia, e.g. in hyperparathyroidism or myeloma. The eyes may be a source of striking physical signs in hypercalcaemia, with a marked conjunctivitis due to calcium deposition (Figure 37), which itself may be evident on the limbus (Figure 38). Metastatic calcification can also affect other tissues, such as muscle, skin and blood vessels.

Hypercalciuria

Increased urinary calcium excretion may accompany hypercalcaemia. Hypercalciuria without hypercalcaemia (idio-

Figure 37. *Conjunctivitis due to hypercalcaemia in a 45-year-old man with acute renal failure due to myeloma.*

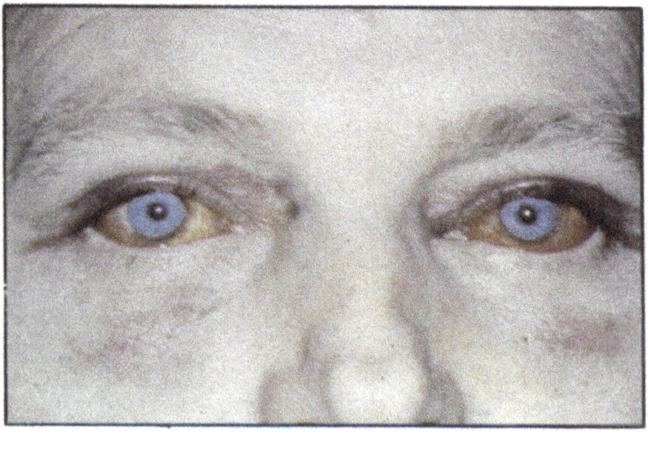

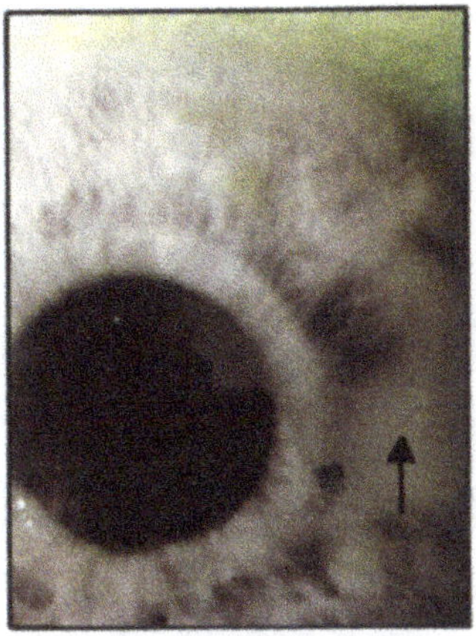

Figure 38. *Corneal calcium deposition (arrowed) in a patient with hypercalcaemia due to hyperparathyroidism.*

pathic hypercalciuria) is a common cause of stone formation. It occurs predominantly in males and is thought to be a result of an increased intestinal absorption of calcium with consequent urinary excretion. A proportion of these cases develop hyperparathyroidism.

Hyperuricaemia

Whatever the underlying disorder—gout, myeloproliferative diseases, status epilepticus or heatstroke—hyperuricaemia can damage the kidney by causing interstitial inflammation, crystal deposition within tubules, and, when prolonged, formation of uric acid stones (only 20 per cent of which are radio-opaque). When the serum and urine levels of uric acid are grossly elevated, acute renal failure may occur.

Gouty patients have the added problems of the associated hypertension and vascular disease. The frequency and severity of gouty nephropathy seems to have diminished over the last 30 to 40 years, and it is now less common to see a patient with gross gouty lesions (Figure 39) and renal disease. This

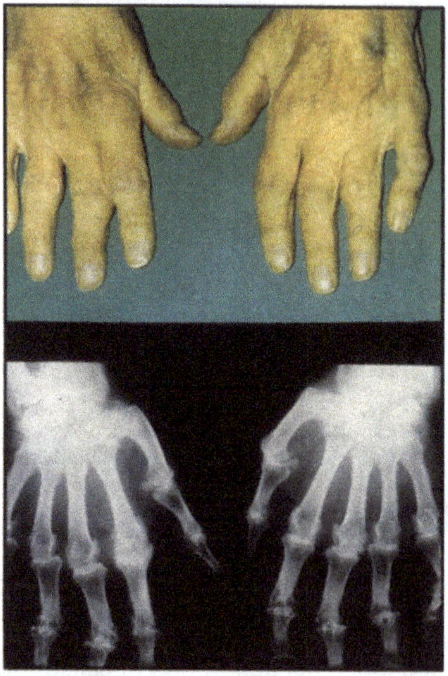

Figure 39. *Hands, with radiograph, of gouty arthropathy in a man with chronic renal failure and gout.*

change presumably reflects improved treatment. Two clinical variants which may present are familial gout, often mild, with severe renal failure in early adulthood, females particularly being affected, and renal failure with mild gout and normal or even reduced uric acid excretion.

Oxaluria and Oxalosis

Oxalate is a constituent of many calcium stones, and disorders of oxalate metabolism cause calcium oxalate stone formation. Hyperoxalaemia occurs secondary to excessive ingestion of oxalate-rich foods and following resection of small bowel which allows excessive colonic oxalate absorption. Primary hyperoxaluria occurs in oxalosis, characterized by widespread deposition of calcium oxalate in the tissues (including the kidneys), nephrolithiasis and frequently chronic renal failure in early life. This condition is due to deficiency of either of two enzymes involved in oxalate metabolism and renal transplantation is unsuccessful despite concurrent transplantation of the enzyme.

Diabetes Mellitus

Diabetic nephropathy accounts for six per cent of deaths in diabetic patients. Proteinuria, found in five to ten per cent of diabetics, is the first sign, appearing on average 20 years after the onset of adult type diabetes mellitus and 14 to 15 years in the juvenile type. The renal disease may progress to the nephrotic syndrome, but relatively infrequently to terminal renal failure, as most patients will die of vascular disease. The appearance of proteinuria is a poor prognostic sign carrying a 28 per cent survival rate at 10 years, and the development of the nephrotic syndrome indicates 30 per cent survival at five years.

The kidneys are destroyed by a combination of glomerulosclerosis, which may be diffuse or nodular (the Kimmelstiel–Wilson lesion) (Figure 40), and vascular disease. There is a good correlation between the development of nephropathy and diabetic retinopathy. Retinal changes precede proteinuria by several years and are invariably present in patients with proteinuria (Figure 41), although not all patients with retinopathy have proteinuria. Diabetes mellitus may also cause renal damage by leading to papillary necrosis, pyelonephritis (although this is now disputed), acute renal failure due to fluid and electrolyte loss in diabetic ketosis, and neurogenic bladder dysfunction.

Diabetes Insipidus

Partial or complete lack of antidiuretic hormone (ADH) causes marked polyuria and polydipsia which can be profound enough to lead to death from dehydration. Diabetes insipidus is caused by cerebral tumours (Figure 42),

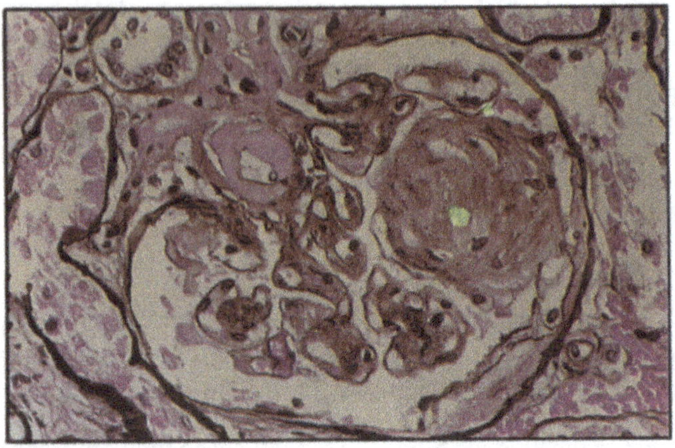

Figure 40. *Diabetic nodular glomerulosclerosis with hyaline material in afferent and efferent arterioles (silver and H and E stain, × 250).*

Figure 41. *Exudates and haemorrhages in fundus of a patient with diabetes mellitus and chronic renal failure.*

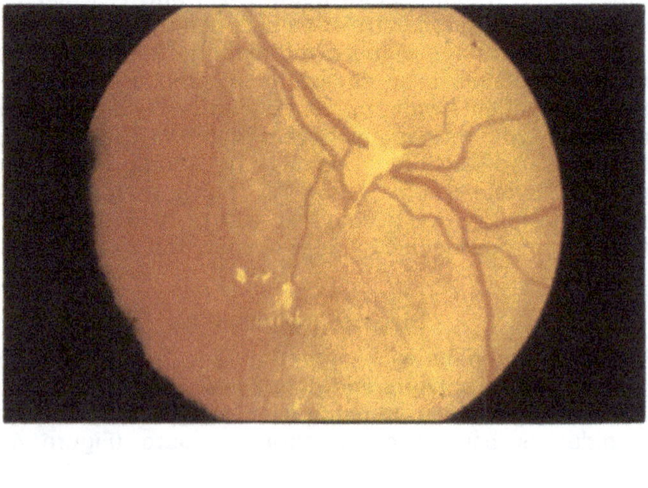

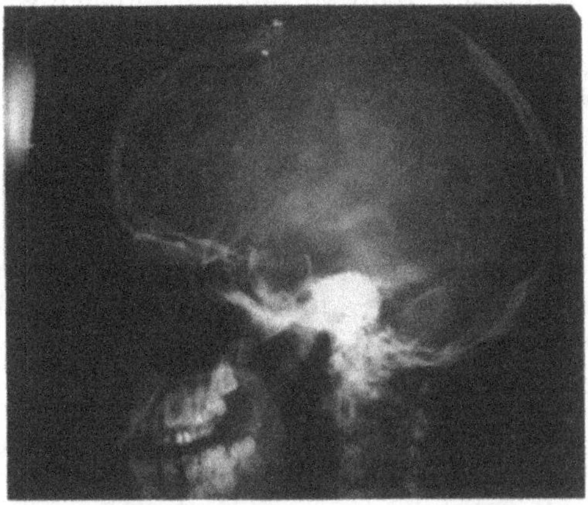

Figure 42. *Radiograph of skull showing enlargement of pituitary fossa due to a craniopharyngioma in a patient who presented with polyuria and polydipsia.*

hypophysectomy, trauma, granulomata, vascular disease affecting the pituitary, infections (e.g. meningitis), as well as an idiopathic form usually commencing in childhood. It may occur in a patient with other effects of hypopituitarism.

A second type of diabetes insipidus is the nephrogenic form, in which there is no ADH deficiency, but the renal tubules are unresponsive to the hormone. This may be acquired with various parenchymal renal diseases such as amyloid and myeloma, through extrinsic influences such as drugs (e.g. lithium), as a result of hypercalcaemia and hypokalaemia, or it may be congenital. The nephrogenic form does not respond to vasopressin.

Compulsive water drinking is differentiated from diabetes insipidus by the normal or raised serum osmolality in the latter compared to the low value in the former.

Inappropriate ADH Secretion

ADH secretion in excess of that required by the intravascular osmolality or volume results in water retention with hyponatraemia and reduced serum osmolality which may result in severe fits, coma and death. ADH is secreted as an ectopic hormone by tumours, the commonest of which is carcinoma of the bronchus, and in association with pulmonary infections and diseases of the central nervous system.

Phaeochromocytoma

Ten per cent of phaeochromocytomas are malignant and they usually occur in the adrenals (Figure 43), but they may occur in other sites, e.g. pre-aortic and pre-iliac vessels, bladder, vagina and rectum. The classic history of paroxysmal hypertension with headaches and agitation is not always present; phaeochromocytomas can cause a sustained hypertension and may also be associated with periods of hypotension.

Conn's Syndrome

Excess aldosterone secretion by an adrenal adenoma leads to hypertension caused by sodium retention. The other

Figure 43. *Tomogram of IVU showing phaeochromocytoma of left adrenal in a 44-year-old man with paroxysmal hypertension.*

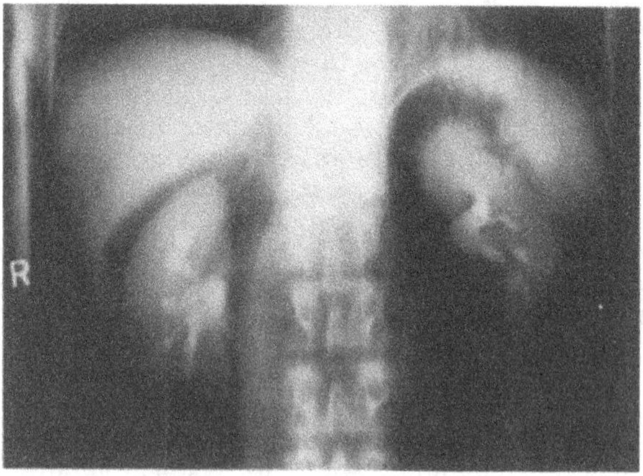

important effect, a helpful diagnostic clue, is a hypokalaemia unresponsive to ingestion of potassium supplements.

Excess or Deficient Glucocorticoids

However excess glucocorticoid secretion arises—by steroid administration, from adrenal adenoma or carcinoma, from excess pituitary ACTH production, or ectopic ACTH—hypertension usually follows. Chronic glucocorticoid deficiency (Addison's disease) results in hyperkalaemia with uraemia, and acute deficiency is often associated with acute renal failure.

Hypothyroidism

Hypothyroidism has been quoted as a rare cause of nephrotic syndrome. More importantly hypothyroidism can cause reversible diminution of glomerular filtration rate and hyponatraemia.

Liver Disease

Hepatic dysfunction affects the kidneys in several ways:

1. Acute renal failure develops in patients with liver damage either because the cause can affect both organs (e.g. carbon tetrachloride poisoning) or because there are reversible effects on renal function in liver failure.

2. Renal tubular defects occur in chronic hepatitis and primary biliary cirrhosis.

3. Hepatic cirrhosis is associated with a glomerulonephritis which is notable for the frequent finding of IgA in the glomeruli.

Evidence of renal disease and liver disease may develop when both organs are affected by the same process, e.g. amyloid (Figure 44).

Fabry's Disease (Angiokeratoma Corporis Diffusum)

Glycosphingolipids accumulate in the body as a result of an

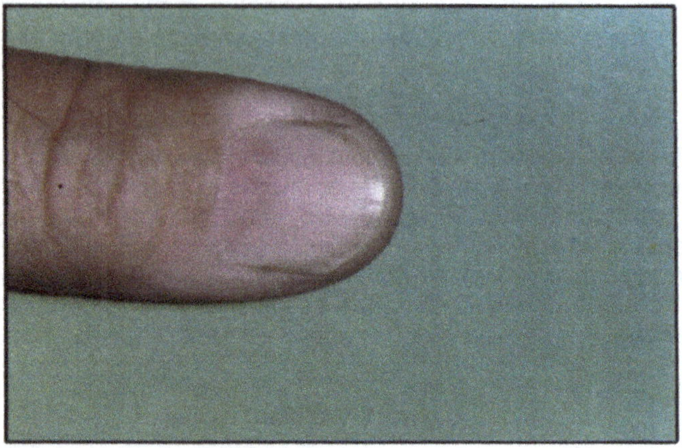

Figure 44. *Leuconychia and purple lunula in a patient with chronic renal failure and liver failure due to amyloidosis.*

X-linked enzyme deficiency. Patients have a distinctive rash of red–purple papules (Figure 45), corneal dystrophy, premature coronary and cerebral arterial disease, and renal insufficiency. The natural history of the renal disease is terminal renal failure in middle age. Transplantation has achieved some success in altering the basic abnormality.

Tubular Disorders

A variety of abnormalities, many of which are hereditary, affect the renal tubules, either as a primary defect in the tubules themselves or because the tubules are involved in a generalized disease also affecting other organs, e.g. cystinosis.

The Fanconi Syndromes

The Fanconi syndromes are a diverse group of diseases characterized by proteinuria, glycosuria, aminoaciduria, hyperphosphaturia, tubular acidosis, potassium loss and failure to concentrate the urine. Clinically they are conveniently considered as three types: associated with cys-

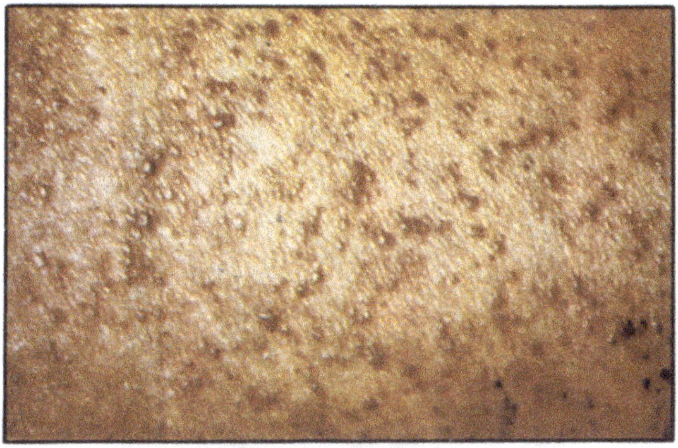

Figure 45. *Skin lesions of Fabry's disease.*

tinosis, without cystinosis, and secondary to a variety of metabolic disorders.

Cystinosis (Lignac–Fanconi syndrome). This metabolic disorder of unknown aetiology is inherited as an autosomal recessive with a gene frequency of 1:200. Cystine is deposited in all tissues, including the kidney where it is responsible for tubular defects and eventual renal failure. The disease presents in infancy with failure to thrive, dwarfism (Figure 46), rickets, and increased urinary loss of amino acids, glucose, phosphate, bicarbonate, water and potassium. Cystine crystals in the eye cause photophobia which contributes to the characteristic facial appearance. The diagnosis is made by demonstration of the typical hexagonal birefringent crystals in the eye (by slit lamp examination), bone marrow (Figure 47) or kidney. Death occurs from renal failure; transplantation will prevent this, but does not reverse the cystinosis.

Fanconi syndrome without cystinosis (idiopathic). The idiopathic form rarely progresses to renal failure; otherwise its effects are similar to those described above.

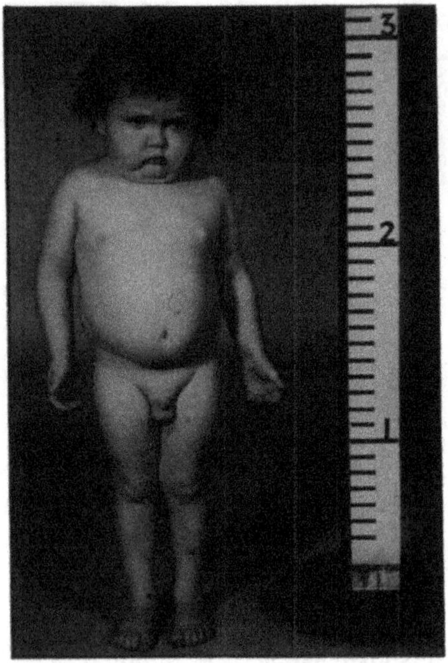

Figure 46. *Dwarfism in a seven-year-old boy with cystinosis and chronic renal failure.*

Secondary Fanconi syndromes. Secondary Fanconi syndromes occur in such conditions as heavy metal poisoning, use of outdated tetracycline, galactosaemia, glycogen storage disease and Wilson's disease (Figure 48), in which there is the added abnormality of excess urinary copper excretion. Treatment with penicillamine in Wilson's disease reverses the tubular defects.

Renal Tubular Acidosis

Defective renal acidification arises either through failure of the distal nephron to maintain an appropriate hydrogen ion concentration (distal, classic, type I) or through impaired

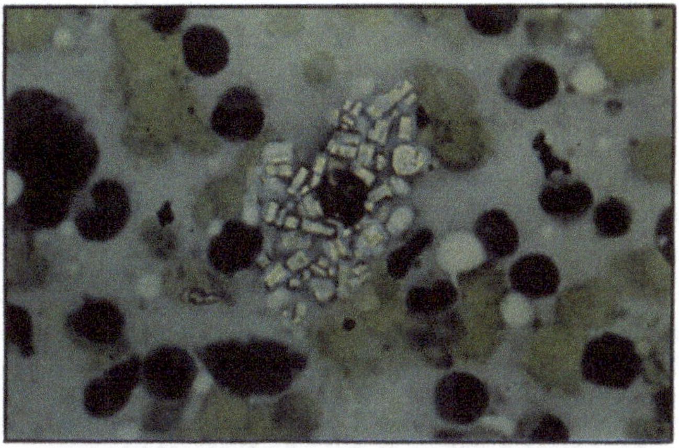

Figure 47. *Cystine crystals in bone marrow in a patient with cystinosis.*

Figure 48. *Kayser–Fleischer ring in patient with Wilson's disease.*

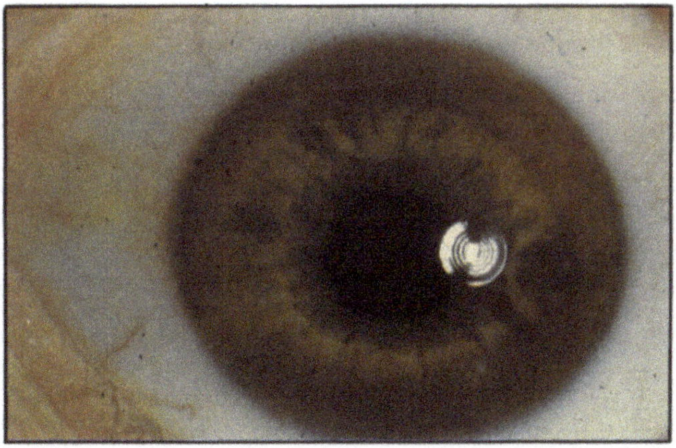

bicarbonate reabsorption in the proximal tubule (proximal, type II). Either form may occur as a primary disease or secondarily, e.g. sickle cell disease, primary biliary cirrhosis, amphotericin B (type 1), myeloma and cystinosis (type 2), when other defects occur, viz. aminoaciduria, glycosuria and phosphaturia. Potassium loss causes weakness, and calcium and phosphate loss cause stones, nephrocalcinosis, osteomalacia and failure to grow.

Cystinuria

Transport defects, which also affect the small intestine, allow excess urinary loss of lysine, arginine, ornithine and cystine. Only cystinuria is significant as stone formation results. Cystine stones are characteristically less opaque than calcium stones and are homogeneous radiologically (Figure 49). Cystinuria is transmitted as an autosomal recessive.

Pseudohypoparathyroidism

Failure of the tubules to respond to parathyroid hormone results in hypocalcaemia, hyperphosphataemia and raised alkaline phosphatase. Patients are usually mentally retarded, short, obese, with short metacarpals, metatarsals or both (Figure 50), and dystrophic nails. Calcification of the basal ganglia is a common finding. Tetany and cramps occur due to the hypocalcaemia. A condition with similar clinical features but with normal serum calcium and phosphate levels is called pseudopseudohypoparathyroidism.

Nephrogenic Diabetes Insipidus

(See page 39.)

Bartter's Syndrome

This term describes patients with hypokalaemia, hypochloraemic alkalosis, raised plasma renin and aldosterone, but with normal blood pressure, increased urinary potassium, chloride and frequently sodium. Patients are usually children or young adults and present with polydipsia, polyuria, constipation, muscle weakness and cramps, and tetany. Children exhibit failure to thrive. Renal biopsy characteristically shows hypertrophy of the juxtaglomerular apparatus.

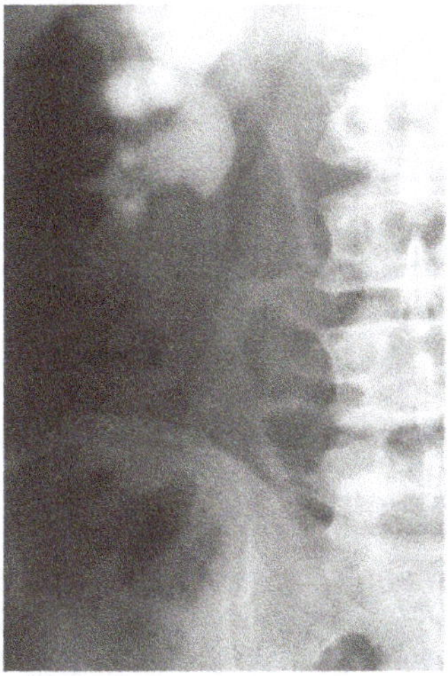

Figure 49. *Plain abdominal radiograph showing opaque homogeneous cystine stones.*

Figure 50. *Digital shortening in pseudohypoparathyroidism.*

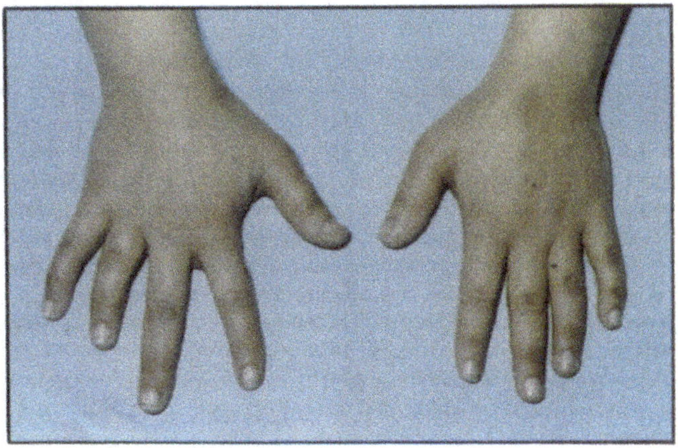

7. Immunological Disorders

The developments in immunology during the last decade have transformed our ideas, but have to a lesser extent affected the management in two areas of renal disease—transplantation and glomerulonephritis. Transplantation is discussed in another book in this series (*Acute and Chronic Renal Failure*, Boulton-Jones 1981). The remainder of this section will be devoted to glomerulonephritis.

Most cases of glomerulonephritis follow from one of two types of immune disorder. In the first, circulating immune complexes (antigen and antibody) are deposited in the kidney and there set in train inflammation, e.g. by activating complement. In the second an antibody is directed against the basement membrane of the kidney.

Immune Complexes

Immune complex damage is thought to be responsible for most human cases of nephritis. Direct evidence (elution of antigen and antibody to it from the glomeruli) for this is lacking in most individual instances, the diagnosis usually being made on the histological demonstration of deposits and the immunofluorescent appearance, with occasionally the addition of a positive test alleged to demonstrate immune complexes in the circulation.

Immune complex glomerulonephritis occurs in two groups clinically—primary, in which the nephritis occurs alone without involvement of other organs, and secondary, in which the nephritis occurs in the setting of a systemic disease.

Primary Immune Complex Glomerulonephritis

Patients may present with any of the clinical features of nephritis, from symptomless proteinuria to the nephrotic syndrome with acute renal failure (Figure 51), and the histological changes may be any of those described in *Renal Glomerular Disease*—another book in this series (Sharpstone and Trafford 1981). In other words, one can rarely be confident on clinical grounds alone of the precise glomerular abnormality in a patient with nephritis. There are certain exceptions, such as the patient with recurrent haematuria with preceding sore throats and colds, 66 per cent of whom have IgA/IgG disease, or the adult with a rapid onset of an

Figure 51. *Oedematous face of patient with nephrotic syndrome.*

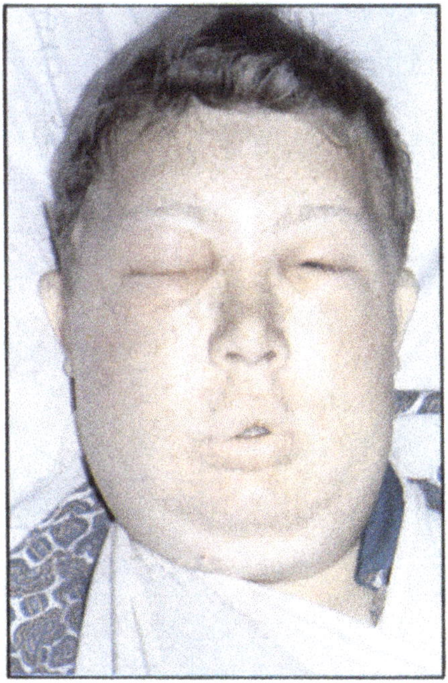

illness proceeding to oliguric–anuric acute renal failure, who is likely to have rapidly progressive crescentic nephritis. Patients with the dense deposit type of mesangiocapillary glomerulonephritis have a rare association with partial lipodystrophy (Figure 52), although not all patients with this strange affliction have nephritis. Another pointer to mesangiocapillary glomerulonephritis is an anaemia greater than would be anticipated from the degree of renal failure.

Figure 52. *Partial lipodystrophy affecting face in a patient with dense-deposit mesangiocapillary glomerulonephritis.*

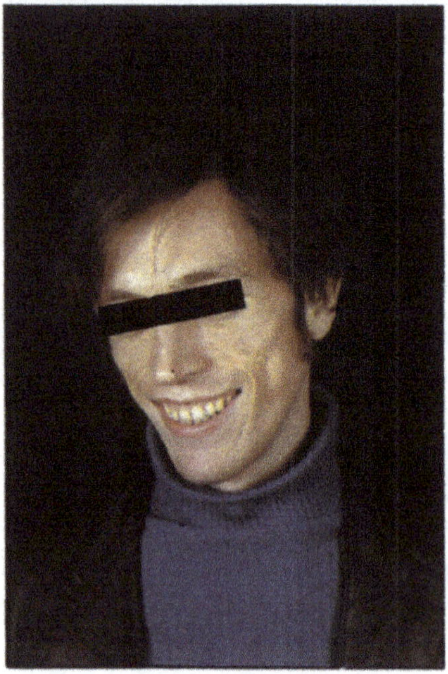

In focal glomerulosclerosis xanthomata may develop due to the very high serum cholesterol levels (Figure 53).

Secondary Immune Complex Glomerulonephritis

Systemic lupus erythematosus (SLE). The reported frequency of renal involvement in SLE depends on the thoroughness with which the diagnosis is prosecuted. Renal biopsy specimens show nephritis in up to 90 per cent of patients, including some who have neither haematuria nor proteinuria. Using urinary abnormalities alone as a means of diagnosis, the proportion of affected patients is 35 to 40 per cent.

The disease is commoner in women than men (10:1), and the glomerulonephritis may present with any of haematuria and/or proteinuria, nephrotic syndrome, and renal failure. The commonest clinical accompaniments in patients with renal disease are a rash (Figures 54 and 55) and arthralgia; retinal involvement may be seen (Figure 56). The glomeruli exhibit a range of abnormalities—focal proliferative, membranous, mesangial and diffuse proliferative, with or without

Figure 53. *Xanthomata over elbow in a patient with focal glomerulosclerosis and hyperlipidaemia.*

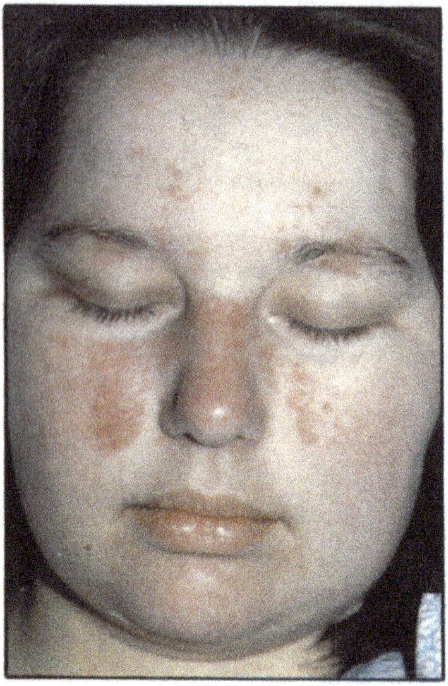

Figure 54. *Facial rash in SLE.*

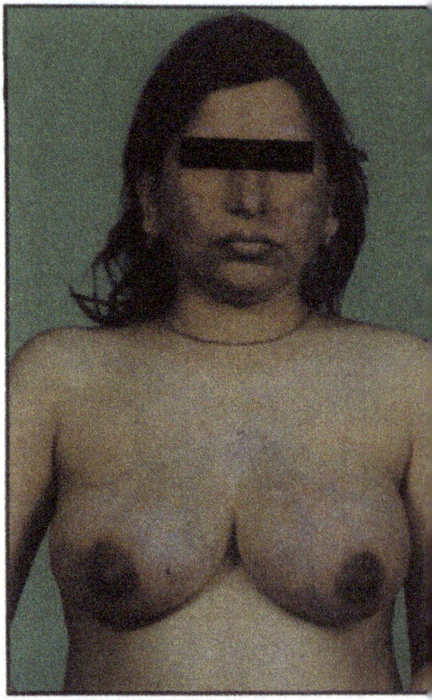

Figure 55. *Rash affecting face and breasts in SLE.*

crescents, and during the course of the disease a patient may change from one group to another.

Recently the prognosis of SLE nephritis has improved; this is thought to be a result of the more frequent use of immunosuppressive agents in management. Five year survival to death or terminal renal failure is now approximately 80 per cent.

Scleroderma. Approximately half the patients with scleroderma have evidence of renal involvement which often declares itself as a rapidly developing renal failure. Patients typically have skin changes (Figure 57) and visceral involvement, e.g. oesophagus. A particular variant is the CSRT

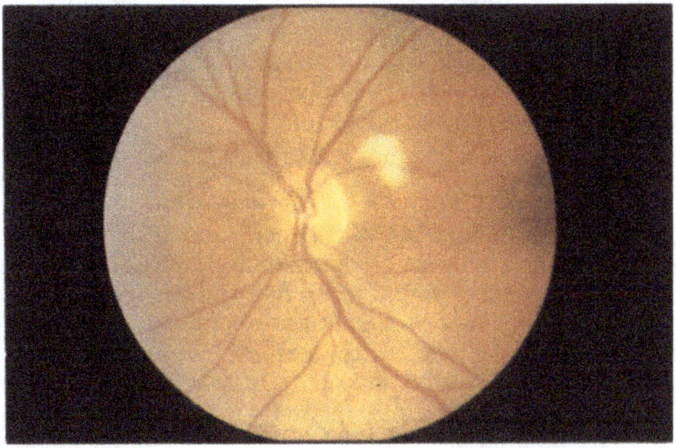

Figure 56. *Cytoid body in fundus of patient with SLE.*

Figure 57. *Fingers of a patient with scleroderma, hypertension and renal failure.*

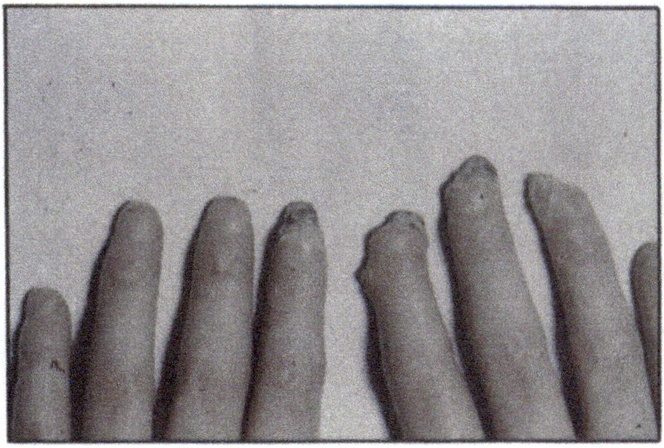

syndrome, in which there is calcinosis, scleroderma, Raynaud's phenomenon and telangiectasia (Figure 58). Severe hypertension is a common feature; it is secondary to the vascular disease of the kidney, which microscopically consists of gross intimal thickening.

Polyarteritis. See page 25.

Rheumatoid arthritis (RA). A reduced glomerular filtration rate is found in a proportion of patients with RA (Figures 59 and 60). Rather surprisingly, since RA is considered to be an immune complex disorder, glomerulonephritis is not a pronounced clinical or histological feature; indeed there is dispute over whether it actually occurs. However, other causes of renal disease do operate, namely amyloidosis, papillary necrosis, interstitial nephritis, vascular abnormalities ranging from an arteritis to intimal thickening of the small arteries, and the complications of gold and penicillamine therapy.

Sjögren's syndrome. Glomerulonephritis or interstitial nephritis may occur as part of this disease.

Figure 58. *Palmar telangiectases in thenar eminence in a patient with CSRT syndrome.*

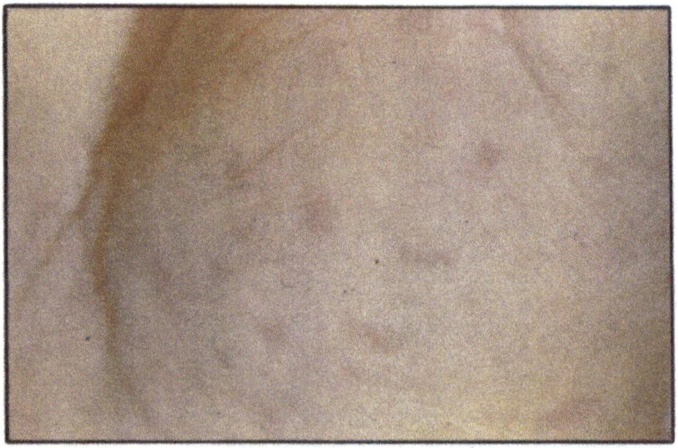

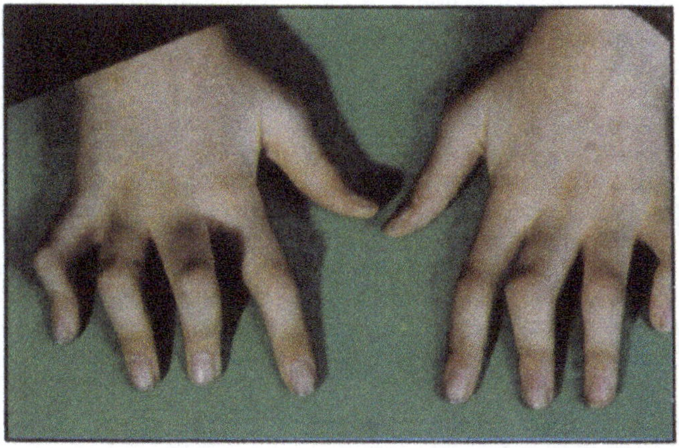

Figure 59. *Hands of a patient with juvenile rheumatoid arthritis.*

Figure 60. *Eye of same patient as Figure 59 showing synechiae.*

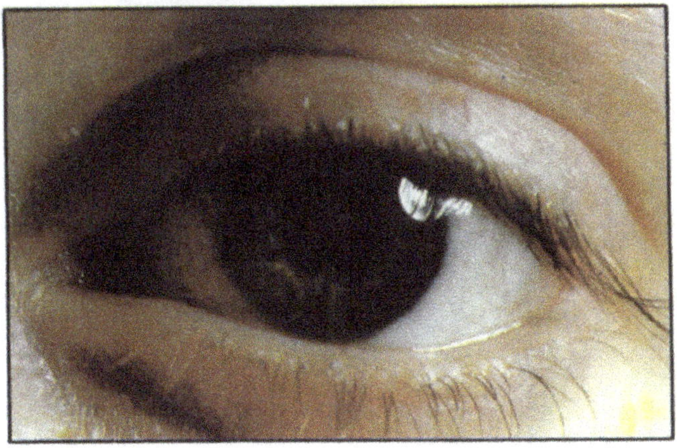

Infective endocarditis. Hypocomplementaemia, cryoglobulinaemia and circulating immune complexes have all been detected in patients with endocarditis (Figure 61). It is not surprising therefore that a glomerulonephritis (Figure 62) can develop in this setting, and its probable immune complex nature is underlined by the immunofluorescent pattern of granular C3 in capillary walls with mesangial IgG and IgM, and by the presence of subepithelial deposits (humps). In addition, emboli from the vegetations can cause infarction.

About 50 per cent of patients with infective endocarditis have evidence of nephritis. In many the clinical effect of the renal involvement is mild, but renal failure does occur. Eradication of the infecting organism, by drugs or by operation, is

Figure 61. *Vegetations on mitral valve of patient with infective endocarditis and glomerulonephritis.*

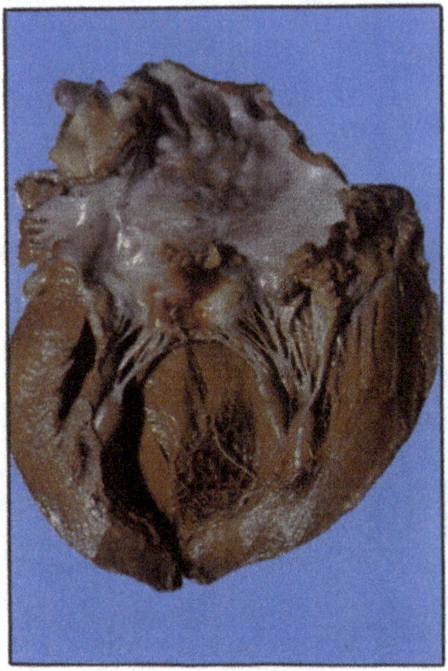

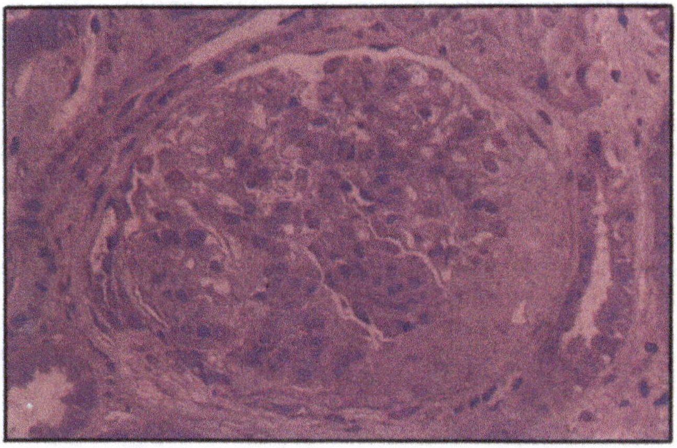

Figure 62. *Glomerulus with three segmental lesions associated with infective endocarditis (Araldite section, toluidine blue stain, × 250).*

frequently followed by improvement in the nephritis, and by an increase in renal function. This exemplifies the alteration in the course of an immune complex disease when the antigen is removed.

Shunt nephritis. Patients with a shunt inserted from the brain to the right atrium or superior vena cava for the relief of raised intracranial pressure run the risk of developing chronic infection usually as a result of a growth of *Staphylococcus albus* on the shunt. A nephritis may follow which is remarkable for its histological consistency in being of mesangiocapillary type. As in infective endocarditis, hypocomplementaemia, cryoglobulinaemia and circulating immune complexes have been found, indicating the immune complex nature of shunt nephritis. Patients with shunt nephritis also show improvement when the infection is removed.

Mixed cryoglobulinaemia. This is a rare syndrome of arthralgia, purpura and glomerulonephritis, characterized by a circulating cryoglobulin composed of IgG and IgM. The IgM of the cryoglobulin is an antibody against the IgG and so is analogous to rheumatoid factor.

Interstitial nephritis. Infiltration of the renal interstitium is seen in some patients with either immune complex or anti-glomerular basement membrane (anti-GBM) glomerulonephritis. More rarely an interstitial nephritis is the main or only histological abnormality, and in some cases the disease seems to be related to exposure to antibiotics (methicillin, ampicillin, penicillin) or diuretics (frusemide). It is suspected that the drugs are responsible for an allergy producing the nephritis, and other allergic manifestations may occur simultaneously (Figure 63).

Anti-basement Membrane Antibody

Antibody to the glomerular basement membrane frequently cross reacts with lung basement membrane; consequently these patients may have lung disease which often manifests itself by haemorrhage either externally or internally or both.

Figure 63. *Lesions of Stevens–Johnson syndrome accompanying interstitial nephritis in a patient who had received penicillin.*

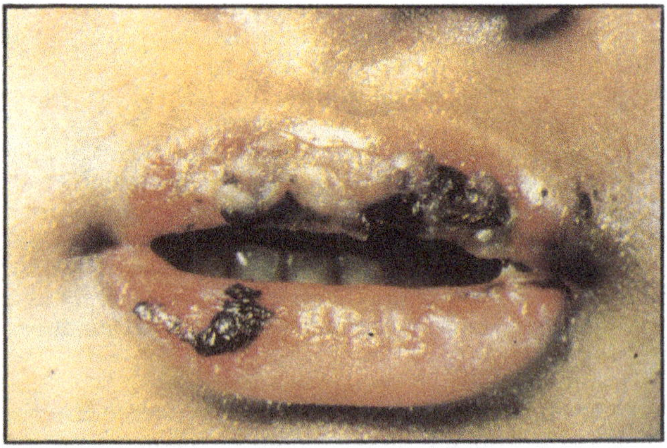

This combination of nephritis and lung disease, first described by Goodpasture in 1919, is called Goodpasture's syndrome. His cases followed influenzal pneumonia during the pandemic of 1918–1919 and it is interesting that many patients give a history of preceding chest infection or, more recently, of undue exposure to hydrocarbon fumes. These preceding events suggest that the antibody is primarily formed against damaged lung basement membrane and then cross reacts with glomerular basement membrane.

The nephritis may present with a clinical picture ranging from a rapid onset of renal failure with anuria to a more indolent course with haematuria and proteinuria. The pulmonary involvement may be symptomless, cause haemoptysis, or produce respiratory failure by intrapulmonary haemorrhage. Diagnostic features are inappropriate anaemia (due to the pulmonary haemorrhage) and signs of lung disease which may be first apparent on a chest radiograph (Figure 64). It must be remembered that patients with nephritis can develop pulmonary haemorrhage from other causes, e.g. thrombocytopenia.

Figure 64. *Radiograph of pulmonary shadowing in a patient with intrapulmonary haemorrhage and acute glomerulonephritis due to circulating antiglomerular basement membrane antibody.*

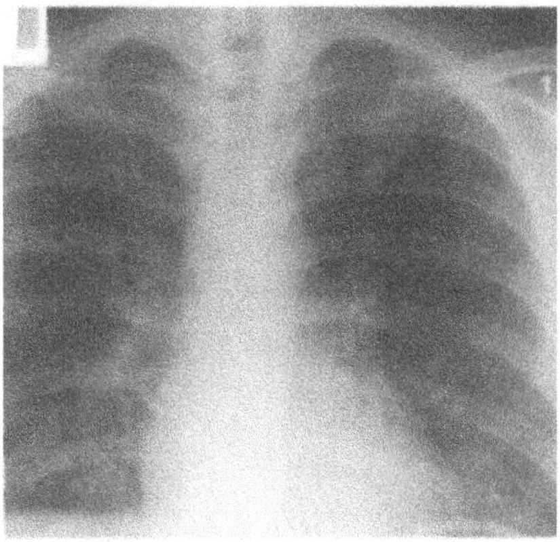

Although rare, accounting for two to five per cent of cases of human nephritis, it is important to make a swift diagnosis, since treatment with plasmapharesis has greatly improved the outcome.

Anti-tubular basement antibodies are even rarer than antibodies to glomerular basement membrane; they have been found in patients with tubular dysfunction and no evidence of glomerular disease, but they also occur in anti-GBM disease and in some cases of immune complex nephritis.

Minimal Change Nephrotic Syndrome

From an aetiological point this nephropathy must be considered separately. It is, strictly speaking, not a nephritis since there is no evidence of inflammation in the kidney. Despite the remarkable response to steroids and immunosuppressive drugs such as cyclophosphamide and azathioprine, there is as yet no convincing proof that it is an immunological disorder. Such evidence is mainly based on the association of minimal change disease with pollen sensitivity and its remission with treatment of the allergy, and its association with atopy.

Minimal change nephrotic syndrome affects mostly children, accounting for 80 per cent of childhood nephrotics and 10 per cent of adult nephrotics.

8. Hereditary and Congenital Diseases

This chapter describes a number of conditions which, although they may vary in their pathogenesis, are inherited or congenital or both. Some hereditary disorders have already been described in other sections, e.g. tubular defects (Chapter 6).

Polycystic Kidneys

Multiple cysts, presumed to arise in the collecting ducts, develop in the kidneys, and eventually destroy them (Figure 65). Two forms of the disease are recognized—adult and infantile.

Figure 65. *Polycystic kidneys (post mortem specimens from a man of 58 who died of chronic renal failure).*

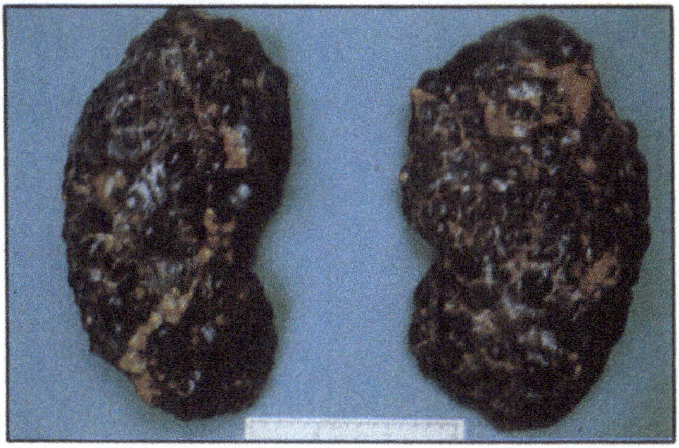

The adult form is inherited as an autosomal dominant; it may also affect children. In about one third of adult cases there are also cysts in the liver, although liver disease does not ensue. Berry aneurysms and subarachnoid haemorrhage are said to be associated. Patients present with the usual symptoms of chronic renal failure and, in addition, haematuria, infection in the cysts, and complaints of abdominal pain and enlargement. Polycythaemia and concentration defects may occur. IVU demonstrates the typical cysts with distortion of intervening tissue.

In the infantile form the inheritance is autosomal recessive, and the liver is always involved with a progressive periportal fibrosis, causing portal hypertension and hepatic failure. Other abnormalities, such as pulmonary hypoplasia, micrognathia, low-set large ears, flat nose and polydactyly (Figure 66), may occur. The condition may present antenatally with a difficult labour, and uterine rupture has been reported. The prognosis is very poor, although milder forms of the disease with longer survival have recently been recognized.

Figure 66. *Polydactyly in a child with infantile polycystic kidneys.*

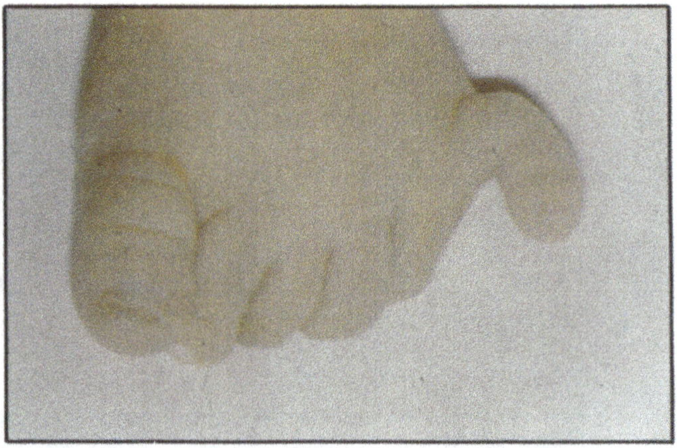

Hereditary Nephritis with Deafness (Alport's Syndrome)

Alport's syndrome usually affects males, who present in childhood or early adult life with macroscopic haematuria, proteinuria and microscopic haematuria, or chronic renal failure. The deafness, which is of the high-tone type, may precede the other symptoms, may be absent, or may occur without the renal disease. There are associated ocular abnormalities such as nystagmus, myopia, cataracts, lenticonus and retinitis pigmentosa (Figure 67).

The inheritance of this disease is incompletely defined. Females, if they have renal disease, rarely develop renal failure; males transmit to daughters but females transmit to both sons and daughters.

Congenital Nephrotic Syndrome

This autosomal recessive condition manifests itself at birth or within the first six to nine months, and eventually proceeds to chronic renal failure. It is relatively common in Finland.

Figure 67. *Retinitis pigmentosa in a patient with Alport's syndrome.*

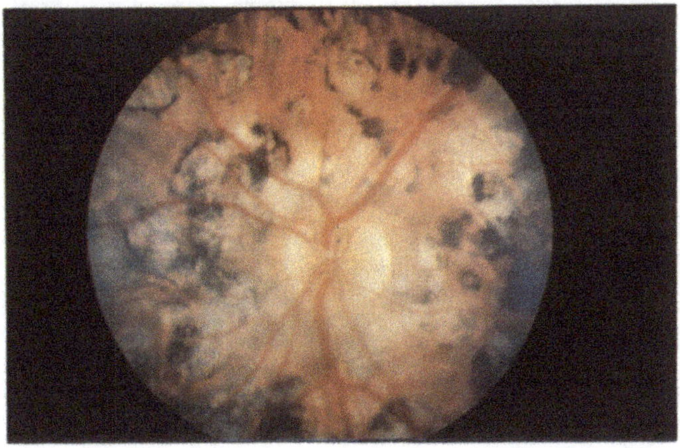

Nail–Patella Syndrome

A defect in the glomerular basement membrane leads to proteinuria, nephrotic syndrome and renal failure. There are associated dysplastic nails (Figure 68), small patellae, and deformities of the elbows and iliac crests. The condition is transmitted as an autosomal dominant.

Gonadal Agenesis (Turner's Syndrome)

The typical webbed neck, cubitus valgus, short stature, mental retardation and sexual infantilism are often combined with renal lesions, such as agenesis, dysplasia, hydronephrosis and horseshoe kidneys.

Nephronophthisis/Medullary Cystic Disease

There has been dispute whether these are variants of the same condition, or whether they differ on grounds of inheritance and age of onset. Here they are described as one. Cysts, derived from distal tubules and collecting ducts, develop in

Figure 68. *Dystrophy of nail in nail–patella syndrome.*

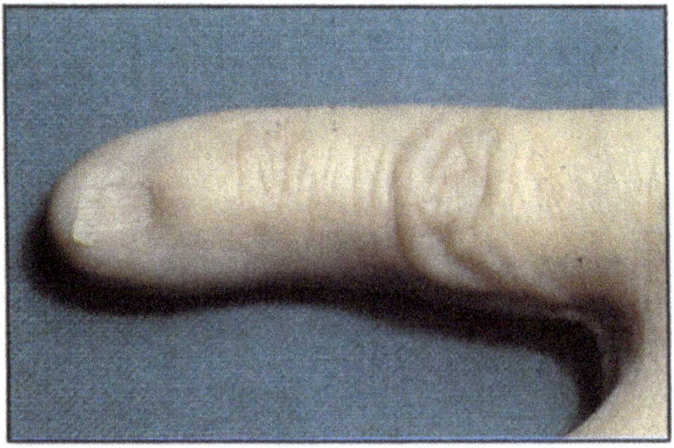

the medulla and corticomedullary region and there is renal cortical atrophy (Figure 69). The disease may present in childhood, usually with an autosomal recessive inheritance ('nephronophthisis'), or in early adult life, usually with autosomal dominant inheritance ('medullary cystic disease'). Patients have polyuria and polydipsia, excessive urinary salt loss and severe bone disease with stunted growth in children; hypertension is usually absent. Retinitis pigmentosa is an associated abnormality.

Medullary Sponge Kidney

Medullary sponge kidney is characterized by cyst formation in the collecting ducts and therefore primarily affects the papillae. The presenting features are renal infection or calculi; radiologically nephrocalcinosis is seen and intravenous urography shows papillary cysts (Figure 70). Familial cases have been recorded.

Figure 69. *Severe interstitial fibrosis with tubular destruction and secondary glomerular damage. Some glomeruli are relatively normal (MSB stain,* × *25).*

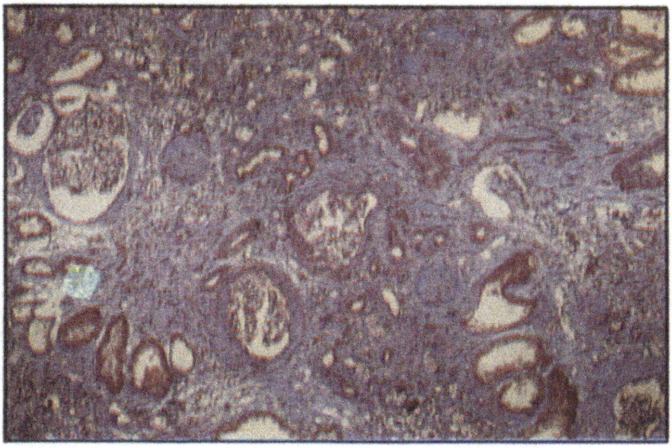

Renal Agenesis, Hypoplasia and Dysplasia

Bilateral renal agenesis, associated with pulmonary hypoplasia, low-set ears, widely spaced eyes and underdeveloped chin (Potter's syndrome) is clearly incompatible with life. Unilateral renal agenesis, occurring at approximately 1:1000, is harmless per se, although putting its victim at increased risk should he/she suffer direct renal trauma, and it may be associated with ipsilateral absent testis, vas deferens, Fallopian tube and adrenal gland.

Hypoplasia (reduced renal mass without developmental abnormality of the parenchyma) may be unilateral, when patients are asymptomatic, hypertensive or prone to renal infection on the affected side, or bilateral when the patient presents in addition with renal failure.

Renal dysplasia (abnormal parenchymal development) may occur with hypoplasia (Figure 71), and is frequently associated with abnormalities of the urinary tract. Dysplasia may be bilateral, with a poor prognosis, or unilateral, when pyelonephritis or hypertension may ensue. The commonest associated abnormality of the urinary tract is ectopic ureterocoele, when the ureter, which drains the upper pole of

Figure 70. *IVU showing medullary sponge kidneys.*

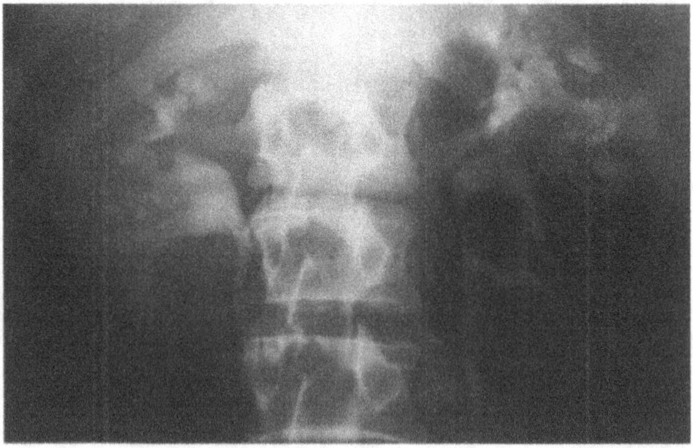

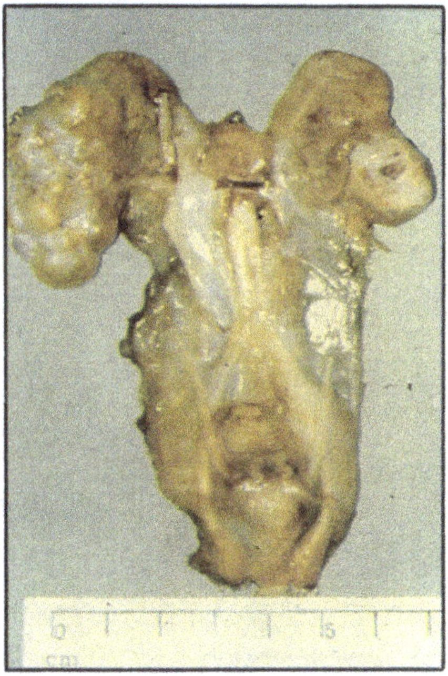

Figure 71. *Hypoplastic and dysplastic kidneys.*

a duplex kidney, opens at its lower end into the urethra below the bladder neck (Figure 72). Hydronephrosis of the upper pole occurs and there may be enuresis and incontinence. Other abnormalities are urethral valves, urethral atresia, and the megacystis–megaureter syndrome in which there is gross enlargement of the bladder and ureters, with reflux and hydronephrosis (Figure 73).

Congenital Abnormalities Causing Obstruction

Obstruction of urinary outflow resulting in hydronephrosis and eventual renal failure can be caused by various congenital abnormalities. Males are more commonly affected by

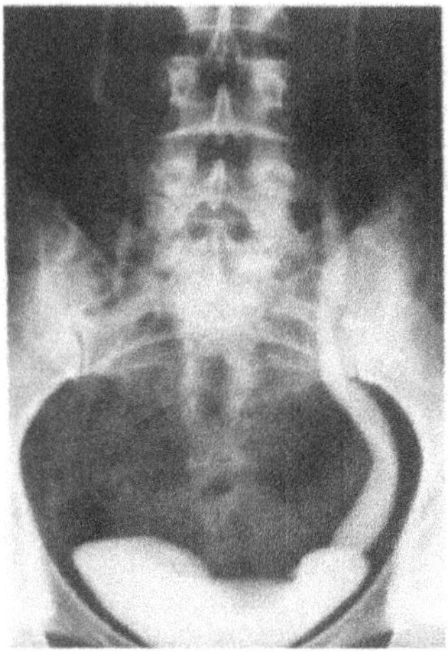

Figure 72. *IVU showing ureterocoele at lower end of left ureter.*

Figure 73. *IVU showing megacystis and megaureter.*

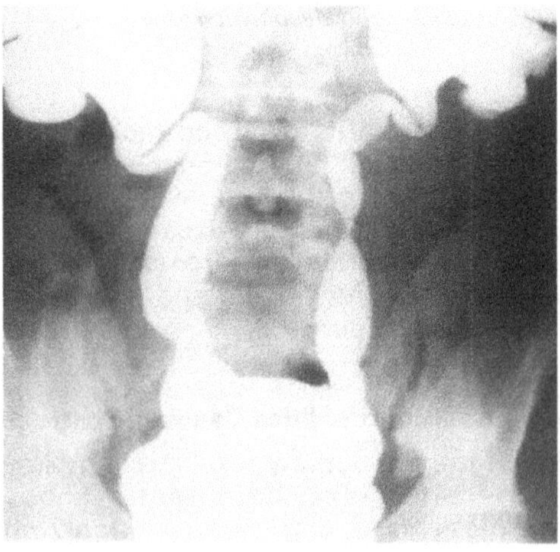

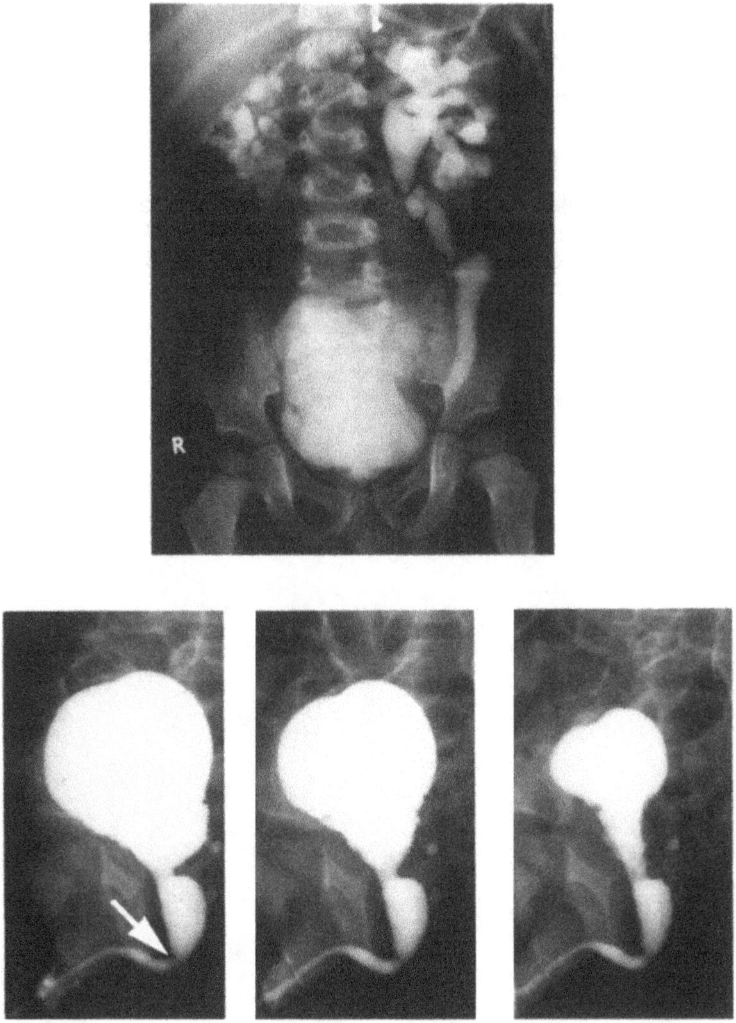

Figure 74. *Boy with urethral valves (above) IVU showing dilated bladder, bilateral hydroureter and hydronephrosis and (below) micturating cystogram showing dilatation of bladder and urethra above valves (arrowed).*

virtue of their predisposition to external urethral stenosis, phimosis and urethral valves (Figure 74). Congenital urethral strictures, stricture of the bladder neck, pelvic–ureteric junction stenosis and neurogenic bladder occur in both sexes.

Vesicoureteric Reflux

This complex disorder can be congenital and familial; it is discussed in detail in another title in this series (*Urinary Tract Infections, Calculi and Tubular Disorders*, Walls 1981).

9. Drugs and Poisons

The drugs and poisons which can affect the kidney are legion and no attempt is made here to be comprehensive. Mechanisms of damage are described with examples.

The kidney is particularly susceptible to the ill effects of drugs and poisons because of its large share of normal cardiac output and the normal process of intrarenal concentration. Furthermore, an important practical effect of renal failure is the increased serum levels of drugs excreted by the kidney with a consequent increased risk of toxicity should the dose not be reduced.

Direct Nephrotoxicity

A direct toxic effect on the kidneys is an attribute of many groups of substances such as antibiotics, e.g. aminoglycosides, polymixins, cephaloridine, amphotericin; organic chemicals, e.g. carbon tetrachloride, trichlorethylene (inhaled by glue sniffers); the elements themselves, e.g. heavy metals; arsine (Figure 75) and venoms (Figure 76), which can also induce renal failure by haemolysis and disseminated intravascular coagulation.

Interstitial Nephritis

Interstitial nephritis may be caused by penicillins, sulphonamides, diuretics and phenindione.

Nephrotic Syndrome

A number of unrelated drugs may cause a nephrotic syndrome, e.g. tolbutamide, probenecid, phenindione and

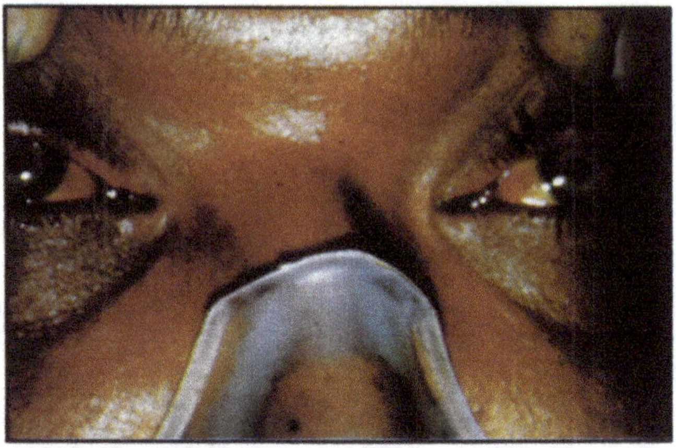

Figure 75. *Pigmentation of skin in arsine poisoning.*

Figure 76. *Infarction of thumb at site of snake bite* (Bothrops atrax), *in a 42-year-old snake collector in whom familiarity bred acute renal failure.*

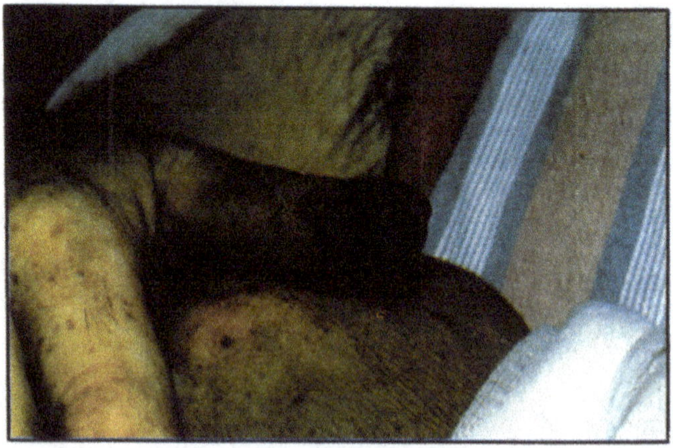

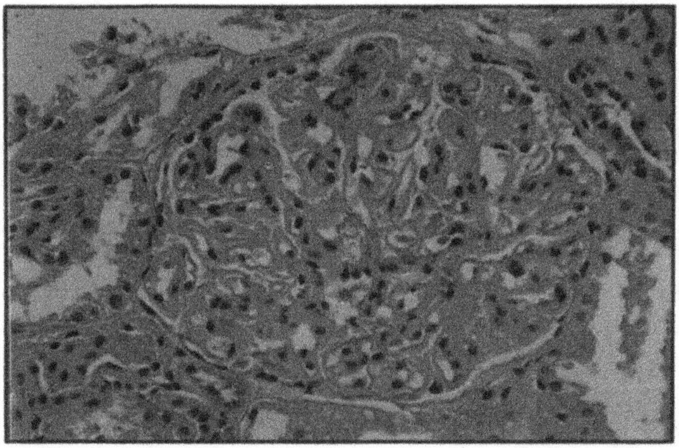

Figure 77. *Membranous nephropathy in a patient who had developed proteinuria while taking penicillamine for rheumatoid arthritis.*

penicillamine. In the case of penicillamine there is an associated membranous nephropathy (Figure 77).

Papillary Necrosis

Prolonged consumption of analgesics can cause chronic renal failure by causing papillary ischaemia and necrosis (Figure 78). Phenacetin bears the brunt of the blame, but salicylates and paracetamol have also been incriminated. These patients have an increased risk of developing transitional cell carcinoma of the renal pelvis.

Fluid and Electrolyte Disturbances

Salt and water depletion causing renal failure may result from diuretics, and any drug which causes diarrhoea and/or vomiting. Hypokalaemia (e.g. from diuretics), hypercalcaemia (e.g. from excess vitamin D) and hyperuricaemia (e.g. from cytotoxic drugs) may each adversely affect renal function.

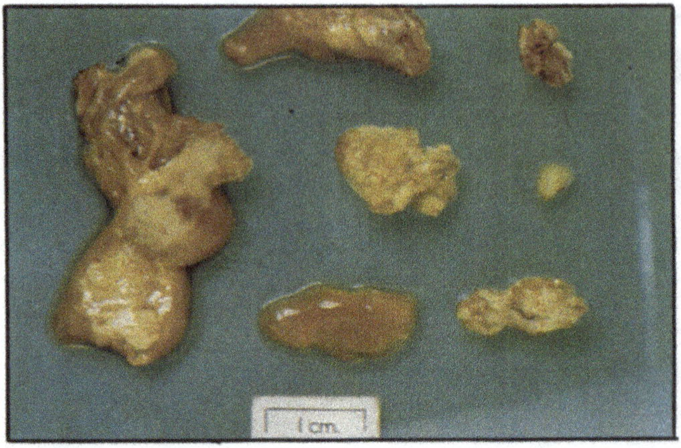

Figure 78. *Renal tissue passed per urethram by a patient with analgesic nephropathy.*

Drug-induced Systemic Lupus Erythematosus

Many drugs have been implicated in SLE, in which renal involvement is less common than in spontaneous lupus. Hydrallazine, procainamide and isoniazid are most frequently involved.

Retroperitoneal Fibrosis

Methysergide, hydrallazine and methyldopa have been reported to cause retroperitoneal fibrosis.

Crystalluria

The less soluble sulphonamides and acetazolamide may cause acute renal failure as a result of their precipitation in the renal tubules.

Anti-anabolic Effect

Although strictly speaking not a direct effect on the kidney, the anti-anabolic action of tetracycline resulting in severe uraemia in patients with chronic renal failure requires mention.

10. Pregnancy and the Kidney

The pregnant woman is at risk of developing several renal complications, some of which may be fatal. Asymptomatic bacteriuria is common, and with it a higher risk of overt urinary tract infection, including pyelonephritis. Obstruction may occur due to the gravid uterus per se, or because there is some fetal malformation, e.g. hydrocephalus.

The most serious complication is acute renal failure, which may arise in a number of ways:

1. Haemorrhage pre- or postpartum.
2. As a complication of pre-eclamptic toxaemia.
3. Following abortion using either operative means with subsequent septicaemia, or drugs, e.g. quinine.
4. As a postpartum disease with disseminated intravascular coagulation, microangiopathic haemolytic anaemia, thrombocytopenia, and marked fibrin deposition in the glomeruli and vessels.

Systemic lupus erythematosus has been alleged to worsen during pregnancy; undoubtedly postpartum exacerbations occur with sufficient regularity to warrant temporary prophylactic increase in treatment.

The prognosis for both mother and fetus when the former has renal disease has much improved in recent years. This reflects the advances in safer and easier control of hypertension, which is the cornerstone of a successful delivery in such patients, assessment of fetal growth, and care of premature babies.

11. Iatrogenic Disease

In addition to drug nephropathy (see Chapter 9), the main methods of substitution therapy in chronic renal failure—haemodialysis and transplantation—have proved a rich source of iatrogenic illness.

Transplantation

Rejection

In a sense this is the commonest complication of renal transplantation, and typically presents with malaise, tenderness at the site of the graft, fever, hypertension, weight gain and diminishing renal function. These are not usually life threatening per se, but occasionally a patient becomes severely ill while rejecting, with high fever and prostration. Rarely in these severe rejections the graft may rupture with the added danger of haemorrhage.

Infection

Infection following immunosuppression, and sometimes transferred with the grafted kidney, is the commonest cause of death in transplanted patients, accounting for 40 per cent in the 1978 European Dialysis and Transplant Association Report. Most occur during the first two months after transplant when dosage of steroids is at its highest and rejection most frequent.

Bacterial Infections

Any species may infect the host, and the commonest are *Proteus* spp., *Pseudomonas pyocyaneas, E. coli, Klebsiella* spp. and *Staphylococcus aureus.* The commonest sites of infection are the lungs, the urinary tract and the wound. Infection of the wound is particularly hazardous when the vascular anastomosis is infected, as sudden and massive haemorrhage can occur (Figure 79). Tuberculosis, which may present as the miliary form, and meningitis due to *Listeria monocytogenes* are less frequent.

Viral Infections

Many patients develop oral and cutaneous infection with herpes simplex (Figure 80), but rarely does the infection become generalized with encephalitis, pneumonitis and hepatitis. Herpes zoster (Figure 81) is frequent and may spread to involve the brain and other organs. Varicella sometimes occurs and may be fatal.

A common viral infection is cytomegalovirus. In most cases the infection is asymptomatic, but some patients develop an illness characterized by a high, swinging fever, yet they have a sense of well-being much greater than would be suggested by the temperature chart.

Figure 79. *Part of wall of renal vein including suture material and related small abscess (H and E stain, × 25).*

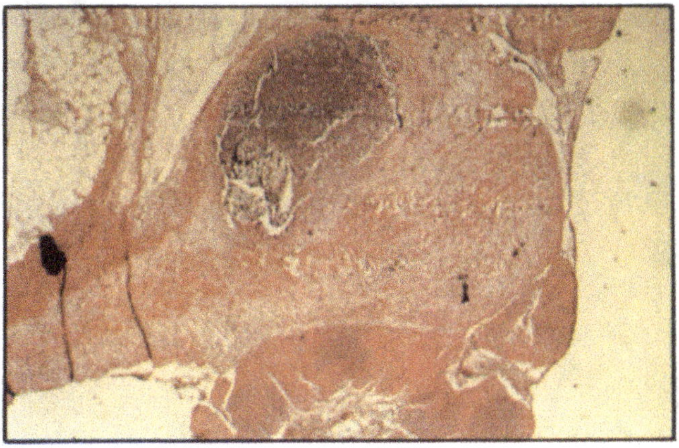

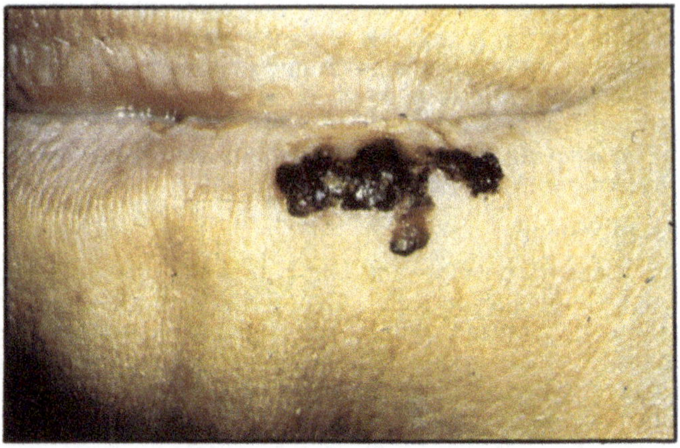

Figure 80. *Herpes simplex.*

Figure 81. *Herpes zoster.*

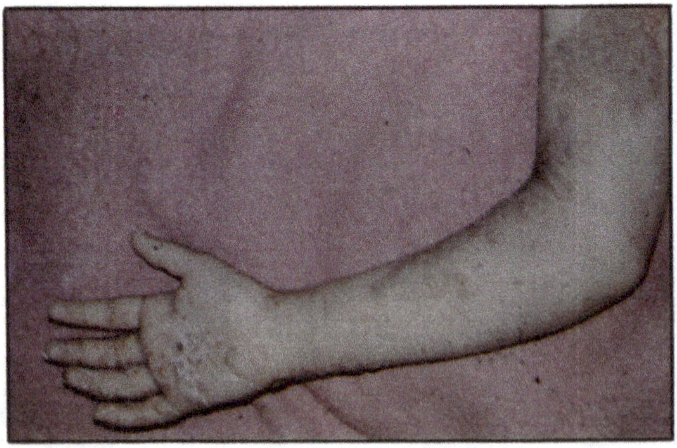

Pneumocystis Carinii

This organism affects the lungs. Usually the patient presents with a fever, cough and malaise, and with progression there is central cyanosis with tachycardia and tachypnoea. Although the chest radiograph shows basal shadowing, the paucity of chest signs is striking, usually just a few basal crackles. Diagnosis is difficult, the only direct proof being histological and therefore requiring a lung biopsy. The rapid response to high dose co-trimoxazole can almost be considered a diagnostic test.

Fungal Infections

Invasion by *Candida* spp., *Aspergillus* spp., and *Nocardia* are lethal complications, with the exception of most gastrointestinal tract infections with *Candida* (Figure 82). The latter is so common following transplantation that it is treated prophylactically. The other sites of infection are lung (Figure 83), when the patient presents with a chest infection or haemoptysis; brain, usually manifesting as a space-occupying lesion; and the urinary tract with symptoms of infection or with the effects of obstruction.

Figure 82. *Oral candidiasis.*

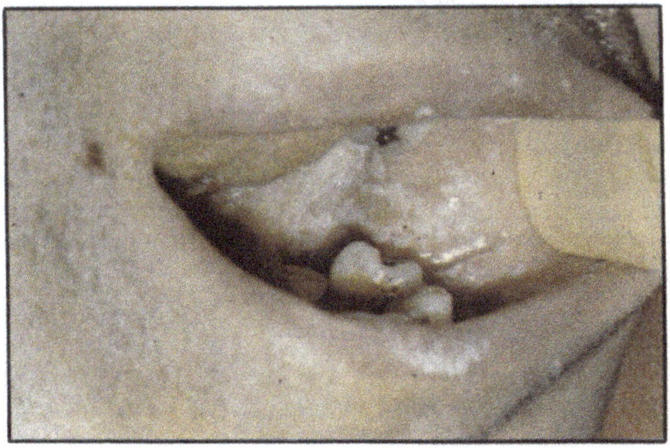

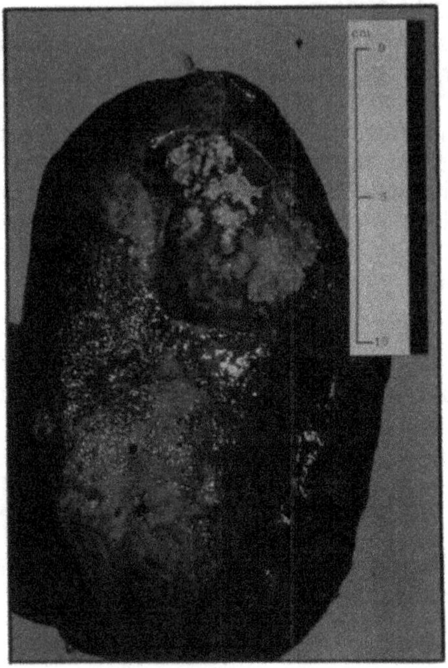

Figure 83. *Aspergilloma in lung.*

Hypertension

Many patients become hypertensive following transplantation as a result of steroid therapy and rejection. A more worrying cause is renal artery stenosis, which may develop at the anastomosis or distal to it through rejection, or tearing of the intima.

Neoplasia

Immunosuppression results in an increased susceptibility to malignancy—in particular lymphomata with a predilection for the brain. Other neoplasms are occasionally seen, e.g.

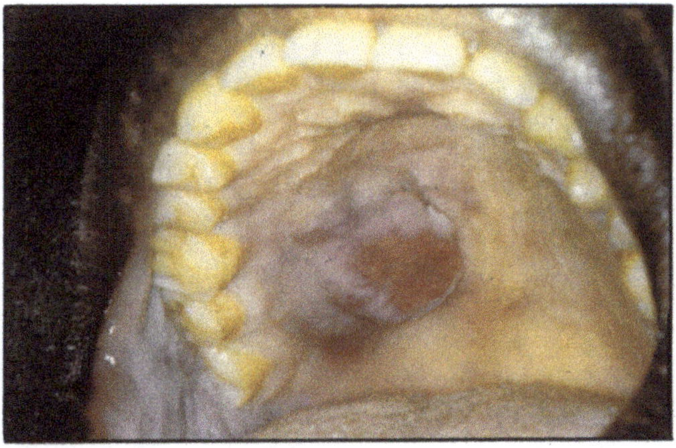

Figure 84. *Kaposi's sarcoma arising from buccal mucosa.*

Figure 84 shows a Kaposi's sarcoma in the mouth of a patient transplanted eight months previously. In Australia squamous cell carcinoma of the skin is the commonest neoplasm following transplantation. The risk of malignancy in transplanted patients is about 30 times that of the normal population, and accounts for four per cent of transplant deaths.

Avascular Necrosis of Bone

The hips (Figure 85) and knees are usually affected, the patients presenting with pain, worse on exertion, and limping. The precise mechanism is unknown, but the condition is related to steroid treatment.

Gastrointestinal Complications

Peptic ulceration with bleeding and/or perforation occurs in approximately seven per cent of patients and accounts for seven per cent of deaths. Steroids are universally blamed despite little evidence; other factors are trauma (operative), infection and ingestion of other drugs.

Acute pancreatitis has also been associated with steroid therapy.

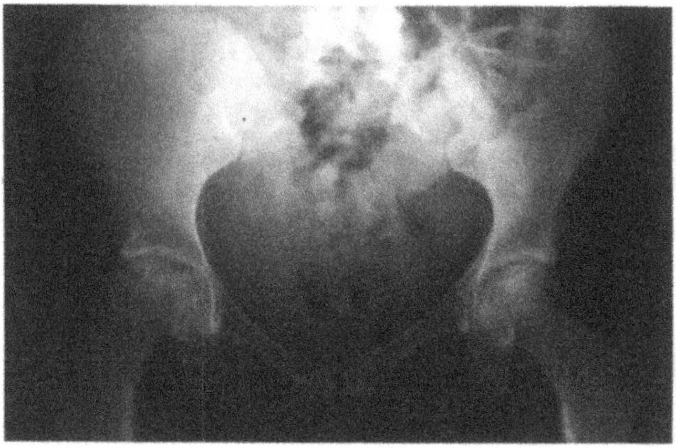

Figure 85. *Radiograph of hips showing avascular necrosis on the right.*

Recurrent Glomerulonephritis

Grafted patients whose cause of renal failure was glomerulonephritis run the risk of developing their primary disease in the donor kidney. The incidence with which this occurs varies with the type of nephritis; it is quite common in mesangiocapillary glomerulonephritis, and surprisingly uncommon in systemic lupus.

Other Effects of Immunosuppressive Drugs

Azathioprine causes marrow suppression and hepatotoxicity occasionally occurs. Antilymphocyte globulin (made in horses or goats) can cause serum sickness, and if the globulin is incompletely purified it may have antibody activity against neutrophils and platelets with consequent neutropenia and thrombocytopenia, respectively.

Haemodialysis

Vascular Problems

The use of an arteriovenous fistula or a shunt makes dialysis patients prone to develop local infection, septicaemia, and even endocarditis. Staphylococci are the usual organisms responsible.

The diversion of blood through a shunt or a fistula can produce ischaemia distally. Symptoms range from paraesthesiae and pain, particularly during dialysis, to frank ischaemic changes in the skin (Figure 86). At the site of anastomosis an aneurysm may develop with the potential dangers of rupture and haemorrhage (Figure 87). As with arteriovenous fistulae at any site, cardiac output rises and a fistula may therefore contribute to cardiac failure, usually with the aid of other factors such as anaemia and underlying myocardial disease.

Bone Disease

See *Acute and Chronic Renal Failure* in this series (Boulton-Jones 1981).

Figure 86. *Digital ischaemia distal to AV shunt.*

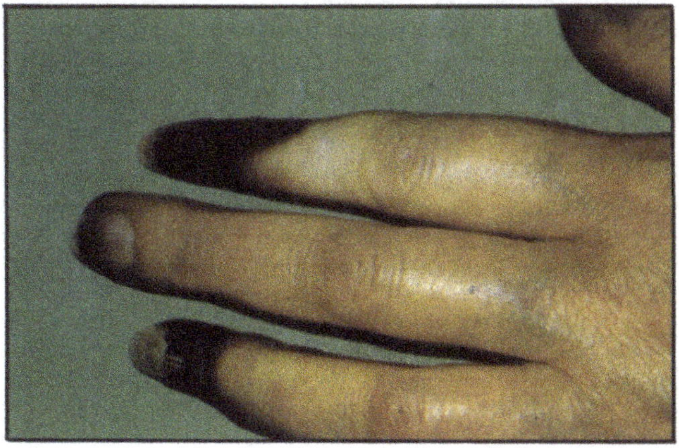

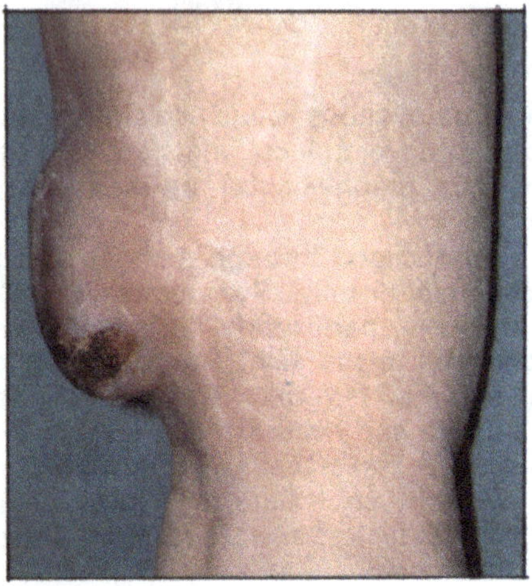

Figure 87. *Aneurysm formation in AV fistula.*

Psychiatric Illness and Dementia

Depression occurs in a high proportion of patients, and there is a five-fold increase in the risk of suicide. Children as well are affected by their new life style, but it is too early yet to say if there are any long-term effects (Figure 88). Dialysis dementia occurs in a small number of patients, who present with amnesia, fits and dementia. It has been related to aluminium toxicity.

Other Complications

The need for anticoagulation in haemodialysis can lead to haemorrhage, and technical failure in the equipment can have tragic consequences, e.g. air embolism.

Peritoneal Dialysis

In the treatment of acute or chronic renal failure the two main complications are peritonitis and protein loss in the dialysate.

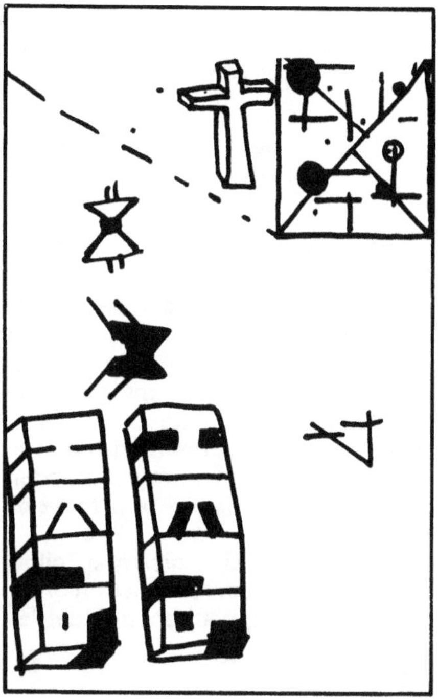

Figure 88. *Drawing by a 13-year-old boy on chronic haemodialysis.*

Radiation Nephritis

Irradiation of the kidneys can produce disease severe enough to result in nephrotic syndrome, accelerated hypertension and chronic renal failure. Unilateral radiation may cause accelerated hypertension.

Percutaneous Renal Biopsy

This procedure can cause haemorrhage, which may require nephrectomy, or can disseminate infection if the biopsied kidney is infected.

12. Obstruction

The many causes of obstruction can have profound effects on the kidney. Acute renal failure may occur de novo or as an added insult to preceding chronic renal failure. Infection is a common complication. Other complications are stone formation, tubular dysfunction, hypertension and polycythaemia (rare). Symptoms range from none to pain, abdominal swelling due to an enlarged bladder, kidneys, or both, the symptoms of renal failure, and those directly due to the causative lesion.

Management of the diuresis which may follow relief of the obstruction is important. Severe depletion of sodium, potassium and water can result, with acute renal failure and circulatory collapse.

13. Self-induced and Imitation Renal Disease

The commonest self-induced renal disease results from drugs or poisons which may cause either chronic damage, as in analgesic nephropathy, or acute damage, e.g. paracetamol overdose or carbon tetrachloride poisoning. Haematuria may be induced by self-infliction of urethral injury and some patients have simulated haematuria by adding blood to a sample of urine. Pseudohaematuria has also been noted to be passive when a relative, usually a child's mother, adds blood to the child's urine.

An amazing range of objects has been presented by patients as having been passed in their urine; Figure 89 shows two examples of pseudostones. Finally, the pethidine or morphine addict who gives an excellent imitation of ureteric colic is well recognized in casualty departments.

Figure 89. *'Stones' brought by two different patients who claimed to have passed them per urethram. Those on the left are gravel chippings, those on the right are date stones.*

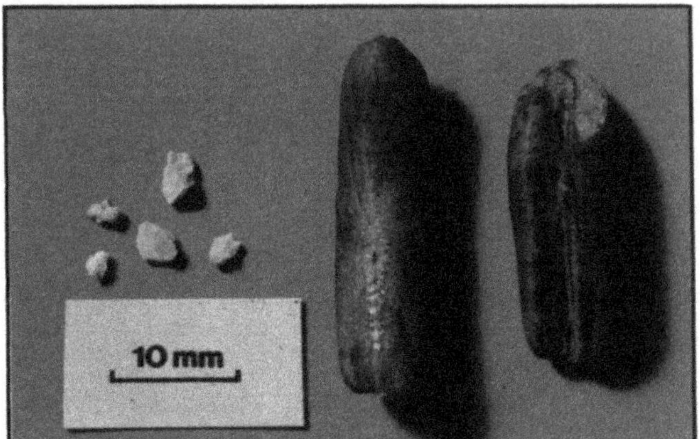

www.ingramcontent.com/pod-product-compliance
Lightning Source LLC
Chambersburg PA
CBHW071355230926
51846CB00002B/566
* 9 7 8 9 4 0 0 9 8 0 6 8 6 *